SEX
HACKS

SEX
HACKS

OVER 100 TRICKS, SHORTCUTS, AND SECRETS TO SET YOUR SEX LIFE ON FIRE

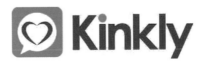

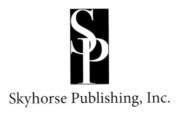

Skyhorse Publishing, Inc.

Skyhorse Publishing books may be purchased in bulk at special discounts for sales promotion, corporate gifts, fund-raising, or educational purposes. Special editions can also be created to specifications. For details, contact the Special Sales Department, Skyhorse Publishing, 307 West 36th Street, 11th Floor, New York, NY 10018 or info@skyhorsepublishing.com.

Skyhorse® and Skyhorse Publishing® are registered trademarks of Skyhorse Publishing, Inc.®, a Delaware corporation.

Visit our website at www.skyhorsepublishing.com.

10 9 8 7 6 5 4 3 2 1

Library of Congress Cataloging-in-Publication Data is available on file.

Cover design by Rain Saukas

Print ISBN: 978-1-63450-574-1
Ebook ISBN: 978-1-63450-979-4

Printed in China

Contents

Introduction

hack *noun* \hak\

A tool, technique, shortcut, or skill that makes a task easier or more efficient, or that solves a common problem in a cleverly inspired manner.

Whether they're for cleaning, organizing, cooking, or making your iPhone perform yet another handy task, life hacks have been helping solve problems in offices, bathrooms, closets, and kitchens for years. Well, we here at Kinkly are all for an efficient life and organized closets, but mostly we're about *sex*, and ensuring that our readers have the absolute best sex of their lives. That got us thinking: with all the handy tips and tricks out there to streamline every other area of our lives, where are the hacks for our sex lives?

After all, many of us really need a boost in the bedroom. According to the Durex Sexual Wellbeing Global Survey, 60 percent of respondents believed that sex was a "fun, enjoyable, and vital part of life," yet only 44 percent of people were fully satisfied with their sex lives. In other words, the vast majority of us aren't getting the sex we want.

Why? Well, our readers tend to tell us that it boils down to three simple reasons: lack of time, energy, and just the simple desire to throw off their clothes and get down and dirty.

But you know what? Sex doesn't have to be one more thing on a long to-do list. It doesn't have to be complicated, fussy, or even messy (unless, of course, you like it that way). With just a little know-how, you can make each and every sexy time—whether alone or with a partner—simple, sweet, and super satisfying. You just need to know what to do to get there.

We wanted to help, so we reached out to the top sex educators, writers, bloggers, and experts we know for their best tips on how to make your sex life better than ever. From tips on sex toys to fun positions and getting in the mood, these sex hacks are designed to simplify your sex life by bringing creativity back into the bedroom (where it belongs!). These hacks are so hot, we can guess what you'll be doing tonight. You're welcome.

A Note about Gender, Sexual Orientation, and Pronouns

We don't know who you are, readers. We don't know if you're gay or straight, if you're male, female, or somewhere in between. We don't know who you sleep with or how. In an effort to be as inclusive as possible, we used a mix of gendered and neutral pronouns in this book. In doing so, we make no assumptions about who you are, how you see yourself, or whom you choose to love. We just hope that some of these hacks will help you hone your sexual skills and enjoy better sex. Because sex is a beautiful thing, any which way you like it.

—*Kinkly Editors*

1: Self-Pleasure Hacks

You might say that we are living in an enlightened age. While masturbation used to be maligned as a health hazard and a dirty habit, something that could lead to hairy palms, blindness, infertility, and sexual perversion, it is now celebrated as a natural stress reliever and a safe means of sexual exploration and expression. Plus, it's a fun and healthy way to pass the time!

Whether you're looking to enjoy a little feel-good quickie or have plans to spend the weekend locked in the bedroom with your favorite sex toy, knowing the proper ways to get off is critical, not only for your own pleasure, but also for your sexual health. In fact, research shows that, particularly

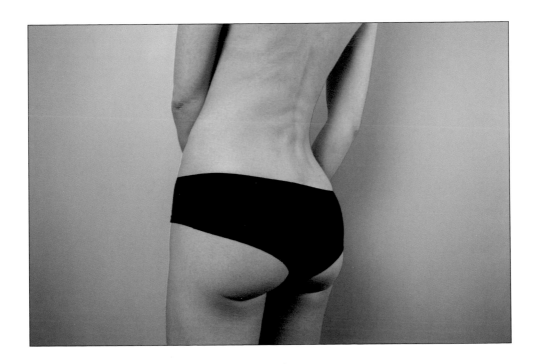

for women, regular solo sessions lead to greater overall sexual satisfaction and more positive views of sex. After all, if you don't know what turns you on, your partner doesn't stand a chance of figuring it out. So, consider your alone time as your own self-taught sex-ed class. While that might sound like serious business, it'll feel like fun—especially if you try out a few of our best solo-sex hacks.

Hack: Let Your Fingers Do the Walking

Sex toys are a great addition to self-pleasure, but sometimes it's good to get back to the basics with the mind-blowing sex tools we already have: our hands. Here's a tip about self exploration from Jenne Davis, the woman and writer-in-charge at clitical.com.

When it comes to female masturbation, you really don't need any specialist equipment, just your fingers . . . Fingers are about as basic as it gets, but they

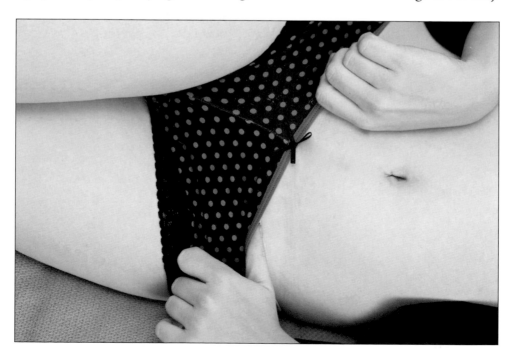

have the advantage of always being handy, never needing batteries, and pro-viding a light or hard touch depending on your mood. Try varying the move-ments of your fingers; circles, long strokes, and shorter strokes all work well. Remember that there is no right or wrong way to pleasure yourself and to include your whole body in the process. Using your fingers can easily put you in the mood for some self-pleasure; run your fingers through your hair, or touch your entire body, rather than simply reaching for the right spot from the get-go. Your fingers are one of the most versatile tools you have in your arsenal for self-pleasure. So why not let them do the walking tonight?

Hack: For Better Sexual Endurance, Use a Masturbation Sleeve to Simulate Sex

Many men have a race-to-finish approach to self-pleasure. And while an orgasm is typically the goal, how you get there counts, especially when you look at masturbation as a practice session for partnered sex. If *that's* over in thirty seconds flat, well, you may have to spend a lot more alone time with your five-fingered friend. A masturbation sleeve, or "stroker," is a great way to simulate sex with a partner and practice maintaining control. Instead of racing to orgasm, work up to taking at least twenty minutes to get there, starting and stopping as needed. When you finally do climax, it'll be much more intense. You'll also have sharper skills to help ensure your next sexual partner leaves the sack feeling satisfied.

Hack: Heat Things Up With a Warming Lube

Sometimes when you get some time to yourself, it's nice to take things slow. A warming lubricant is a simple lube with a spectacular added ingredient designed to create warmth when it's applied. This can increase circulation and blood flow. The more blood you have heading to your pleasure zone, the greater your pleasure will be. Now that's hot! Just be sure to test things out with a little dab first to see how you react. The idea here is to ignite some passion, not set your crotch on fire.

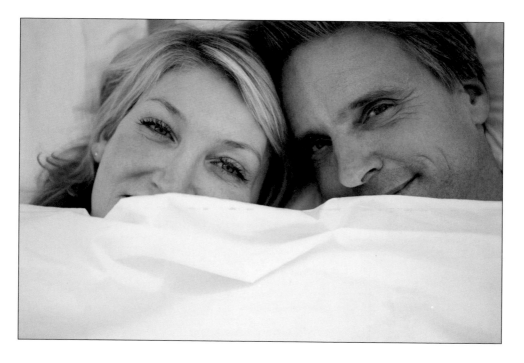

Hack: Do It with a Partner

Masturbation is an important alone-time activity, but isn't *just* an alone-time activity—or it shouldn't be. Sharing a little self-love with a partner can be fun, hot, and provide a great learning experience for both of you. Not only does masturbating in front of your partner provide one hell of a show, it'll also help them get in touch with what you like and what turns you on. It's a very safe form of sexy fun. Plus, since you both know what to do, everyone gets touched the way they want to. So consider turning that solo into a duet once in a while. It could lead to double the fun.

Hack: Turn an Electric Toothbrush into a Discreet Vibrator

Many sex toy novices already have a great vibrator sitting right in their medicine cabinets—an electric toothbrush. This handy device might be designed to make your smile pretty, but it can also keep a grin on your face. Many electric toothbrushes vibrate at a much higher rate than your typical vibrator, creating a different sensation. Plus, you don't have to worry about leaving an electric toothbrush out, or having to explain it to a customs agent while traveling. Some companies even sell special attachments to turn a toothbrush into a personal massager. Don't feel like you need to mix genres here: If you do use your toothbrush to actually, you know, brush your teeth, consider getting an extra one. This clever hack is a best-kept—but well-used—self-love secret!

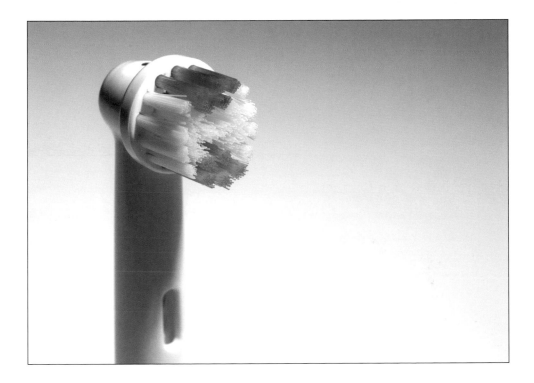

2. Foreplay Hacks

Many people think of foreplay as a preamble—a required formality you have to go through before getting to the good stuff. But the best lovers know better; foreplay is—or should be—a vaunted sex act in and of itself. Think of it like an appetizer; if this first, highly anticipated tidbit fails to impress, how are you going to get excited for the main course? Or dessert?!

Foreplay done right is a beautiful thing. It builds the anticipation, desire, and excitement that brings passion and intensity to sex and makes it truly enjoyable and memorable. Oh, and did we mention orgasms? A study conducted by McGill University and published in *The Journal of Sex Research*

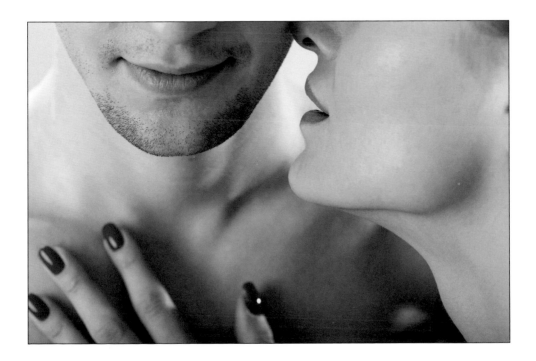

in 2014 measured sexual arousal, buildup, and climax in thirty-eight men and thirty-eight women in a lab. It found that the greater the buildup of arousal, the more pleasurable the orgasm. Now, these lucky lab rats were pleasuring themselves, but whether you're playing solo or with a partner, research shows that the longer it takes you to get to the finish line, the more satisfied you'll be when you get there.

Although foreplay can greatly improve the sexual experience for men, it is crucial for most women. For women, adequate foreplay means they're more likely to enjoy sex, have an orgasm, *and* come back for more. In fact, one study found that 58 percent of women ranked foreplay as the most satisfying sexual activity, and 65 percent wanted their partners to pay more attention to it. Needless to say, if you're having sex with a woman, foreplay will need to be a top priority for you too. No matter your gender, the kissing, touching, and focus on pleasure that comes with foreplay is a great way to show your partner that you care. (*Awwww!*)

These awesome hacks will have you hankering for foreplay rather than rushing through it. Great sex is sure to follow!

Hack: Put Those Nipples Front and Center

For many women, their nipples are a major erogenous zone. They're super-sensitive and they're attached to a part of the body that's often viewed as sexy. Oh, and stimulating them can even trigger an orgasm, or "nipple-gasm." When the nipples are stimulated, oxytocin, one of the body's many amazing feel-good hormones, is released, causing the same uterine and vaginal contractions associated with orgasm. This can send more blood flowing southward, triggering an honest-to-goodness orgasm. Many women enjoy getting the girls in on foreplay, but if you want to take nipple play all the way, start out with gentle caressing and sucking, then move on to creating more intense sensations. Just follow your partner's cues to find out what she likes. Although men's n-zones often go untouched, some men like nipple play too, so it's worth exploring with any partner.

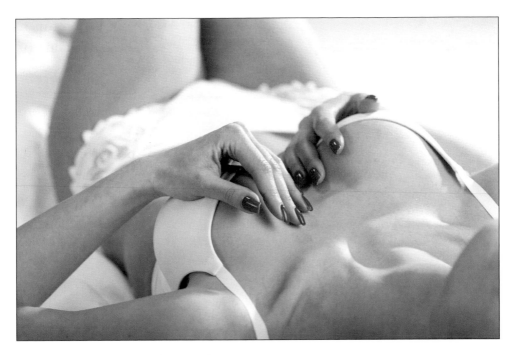

Hack: Kiss Her on the Neck

Kissing is a major part of foreplay; it's the first point of wet, hot, truly intimate contact. But where and how you deliver those kisses really matters,

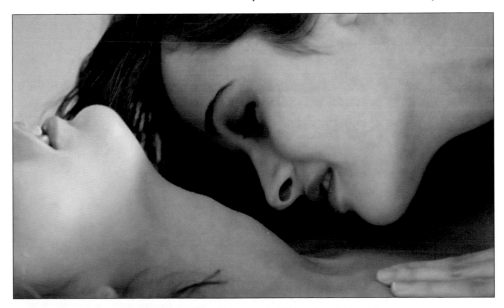

especially for women. Statistics from *The Book of Odds* by Amram Shapiro suggest that 96 percent of women love being kissed on the neck. In fact, it's their favorite spot—after the lips, of course. Try caressing and grazing your partner's neck and shoulders as part of foreplay to tease and tempt, creating greater sexual tension.

Hack: Keep Your Panties On

The teenage you was on to something—pleasuring each other through your clothes can be the sweetest form of sexual torture. Tease and stroke each other through fabric until you can hardly stand it anymore. This builds anticipation. When you finally get to skin-on-skin contact, the results will be explosive.

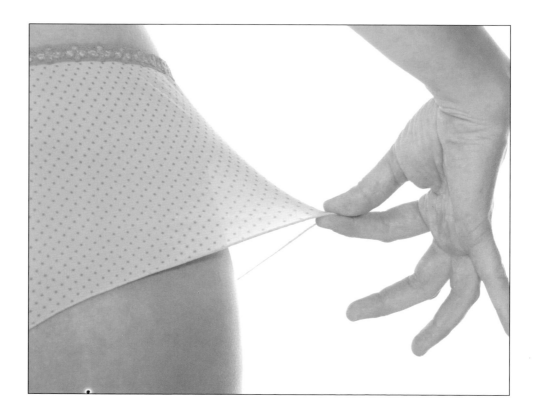

Hack: Scare the Crap Out of Each Other

Want to breathe new life into a long-term sexual relationship? Research has shown that doing an activity with a partner that produces an adrenaline rush can be carried right into your relationship—and into the bedroom. Go ride a crazy-high roller coaster, go skydiving or zip-lining. It may sound scary, but your mind will transfer all that excitement into your relationship, helping you bond in and outside the bedroom.

Hack: Make Dirty Talk Mad Libs

Sometimes foreplay starts before you and a partner even touch each other. Remember Mad Libs? They aren't just for kids anymore. Sex educator and author Ashley Manta recommends using them as a way to ease into dirty talk. Here's her top hack for heating things up.

I like to think of dirty talk as "sexy Mad Libs." Here are some fill-in-the-blanks to get you started:

I love it when you _____ my _____.
I want you to _____ until I _____.
It makes me feel _____ when you _____.
I like the way you _____ my _____.
Feeling your _____ inside me makes me want to _____.
You make me _____ when you run your _____ over my _____.

Knowing what you don't want is every bit as important as knowing what you do want. It is important to communicate your limits to your partner. It is OK to say "I don't want to role play XYZ scenario because it feels uncomfortable to me." Trust your instincts and let your partner know as soon as you realize something isn't working for you.

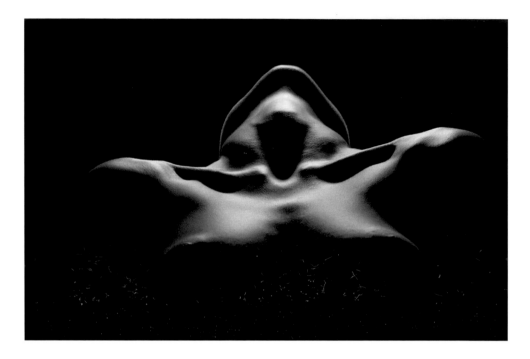

Hack: Use a Flashlight to Light up Your Pleasure Zones

Ever fantasized about a peep show? Here's how to recreate one in your own bedroom—only in this sexual fantasy, your partner gets to touch the goods! Turn off the lights, grab a flashlight, and point its beam to areas of your body where you'd like your partner's attention. You can start with areas like your back, legs, and stomach, and then move on to the neck, ears, and nipples— wherever you'd like them to explore! By the time you're ready to throw the flashlight aside, you'll both be lit up.

Hack: Be Still

We often think of foreplay as a series of movements—kissing, stroking, circling, teasing. Instead, try just laying your hand over your partner's genitals. Look them in the eye, talk dirty to them, and let the pressure and heat of your hand arouse them—and you!

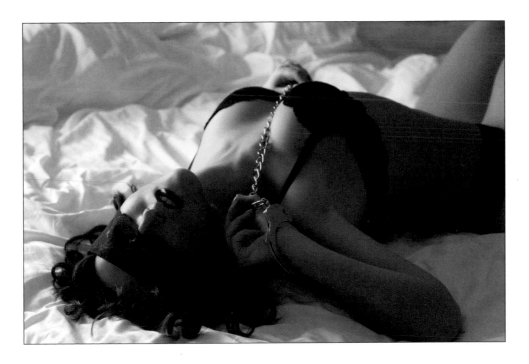

Hack: Intensify Touch by Removing Sight

When one sense is lost, other senses tend to become stronger to compensate. That's the concept behind sensory deprivation, anyway. To put fireworks into your touch, try turning off your partner's sense of sight with a soft, sexy blindfold. This will also provide an element of surprise to what you're doing to your partner, heightening the tension and excitement.

Hack: Incorporate the Element of Surprise

Hot sex in a long-term, monogamous relationship often takes a little work. Once we learn exactly how to push our partner's buttons, we tend to just keep pushing them in the same order each and every time. Why mess with a winning formula, right? Unfortunately, a simple orgasm does not make for great sex. What keeps people coming back for more is desire, passion, and intrigue. This hack comes from Bobbie Morgan, a content marketer for the adult industry and editor in chief at *A Good Woman's Dirty Mind* (agoodwomansdirtymind.com).

Many long-term relationships get boring because people know their partner's patterns, behaviors, and techniques. They fall into them because they're easy and have a history of success.

But "easy" and "sure things" get boring. They're lazy. Surprises come naturally when a couple first falls in love and lust with someone early on in a relationship because people don't know what to expect. Surprises in the long-term relationship take effort because strangers are more motivated to attract and woo a new partner. That same kind of effort should continually take place to keep your partner and relationship happy, sexy, and fun.

Plan a surprise date. Don't give any clues to where you're going until you get there—a couple's massage, a twilight picnic on a secluded beach or at a scenic site at a park. Just go someplace or do something you haven't done before. Send a couple of emails or texts during the day giving your partner brief instructions on how he or she should be prepared for your mystery plans later in the evening.

Try a new position or bring out some new sex toys in bed. Even if it fails, hopefully both of you have a sense of humor and can laugh about it.

Come home and be the seducer or seductress you've always wanted to be, from the moment you step in the door. Or pretend that your partner is someone they've always envisioned themselves being, or pretend they're someone you've wanted to have. (You might not want to let your partner in on that fantasy. It's OK to keep some things to yourself!)

Hack: Stimulate the Sacrum

The body is full of erogenous zones, but the sacrum—the flat, triangular part of the low back just above the buttocks—contains sacral nerves, which are a direct pathway to the genitals. Gently stroke, massage, or lick your partner's

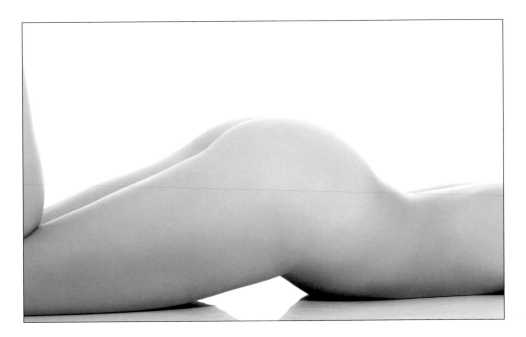

sacrum to help build heat. Some people can even approach orgasm as a result of this type of stimulation.

Hack: Heighten Your Partner's Senses With a Feather Tickler

There's a reason the French maid fantasy is so popular: she always carries a feather duster! Feathers are soft and sensual and feel great against the skin. When you stroke, tickle, or tease your partner's flesh, you're gently stimulating touch receptors and priming your partner for more. You can buy a large, single feather, or pick out a feather tickler at your local sex toy retailer. Try running it down the length of your partner's body, gently tracing around the erogenous zones until your partner is wild for a rougher touch.

Hack: Use Mason Jars to Mix Things Up

Is there anything the mighty mason jar can't do? Pinterest has proved these humble holders as hackable for everything from light fixtures to cocktail

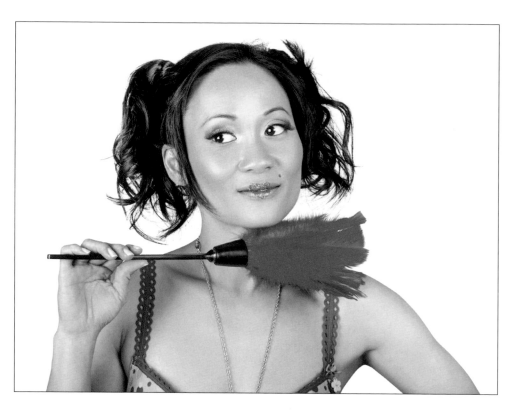

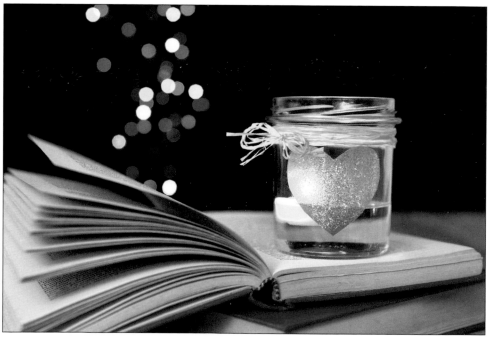

shakers. And hey, once you've decorated those little hallmarks of hipster-dom to your heart's content, try placing them on your bedside table. Jenne Davis, head honcho over at clitical.com, has a great hack for how to make them part of your foreplay.

It might sound cliché, but adding a sex game to your foreplay routine can spice things up. Take two mason jars, a pen and paper, and a pair of scissors. Both part-ners then write down verbs—think "suck," "lick," "kiss," "touch here"—cut them up, and place them in one jar. Then, each partner writes down parts of the human body and places them in the other jar. Take a piece of paper from each jar and let the fun begin! Of course, when the fun and games are over for the night, you can simply put the jars of words away until next time you feel like playing. . . .

Hack: Use Edible Body Paint to Turn Your Partner into a Colorful (and Tasty) Masterpiece

Your tongue has around ten thousand taste buds, and your skin is your largest erogenous zone. Combining the two can make for the sweetest, sexi-est sensation-play ever. And while drizzling your love in whipped cream and chocolate can be a fun and tasty adventure, it also tends to get pretty sticky. Edible body paints offer all sorts of fun opportunities, with much less mess. Use different colors and flavors to write naughty messages on your partner's body, or have your partner "clothe" your most sensitive areas in paint—then ask to have it licked right off.

Hack: Follow Your Nose

Maybe you like to light candles or incense to get your sexy on. As it turns out, these touches do more than just set the mood, especially when certain libido-boosting scents are used. The smell of vanilla has been shown to boost testosterone and libido in men, but according to a 2010 study conducted by Alan Hirsch of the Smell and Taste Research Center, the smell of lavender

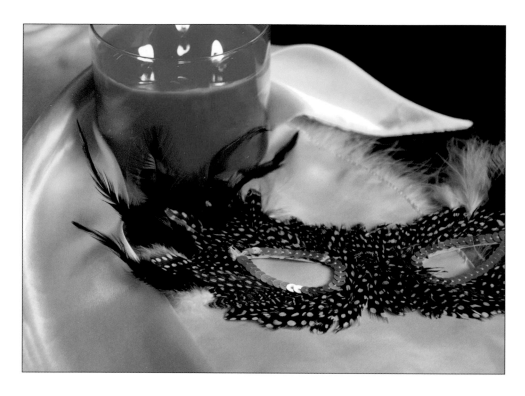

and pumpkin pie are tops at boosting penile blood flow. Licorice and dough-nuts are high on the list as well. Maybe there's a reason why so many people refer to sex as dessert!

Hack: For Hotter Sex, Warm up First

Sex has been proven to be a legitimate workout, but if you really want to be hardcore, you could work out before sex. Not only will you feel hot, healthy, and confident in your body, you'll also be priming yourself for a bit of post-workout, not-so-cooldown, at least according to this hack from genderqueer porn star Jiz Lee.

This sex hack is for couples looking for the perfect full-body experience. Squeeze in a short run or a brisk walk before getting down. The key here is to keep it on

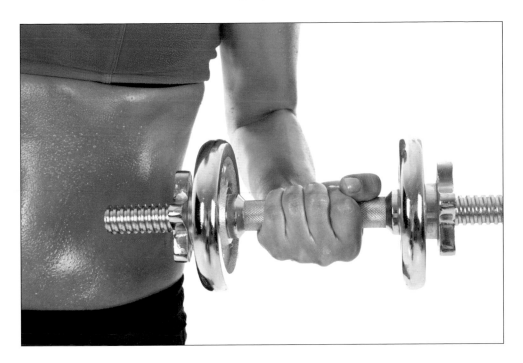

the quick side. (Don't worry, you'll have time to build up a sweat later . . .) Go on a twenty-minute run, or a thirty-minute brisk walk. Then, take a shower (or . . . don't) and burn off the last spurt of energy. With your endorphins on high, you'll be riding on good energy with your partner, and feeling hot and sweaty (if you save the shower for later) or clean and confident (if you rinse off before hand) and will have added an exciting, exuberant tryst into your busy schedule.

Hack: Tap Into Fun in the Shower or Bath

Sometimes heating things up is as simple as turning on the tap. This clean and sexy sex hack comes from Jenne Davis at clitical.com.

Using water as a part of your foreplay routine can add a little spice, and is limited only by your imagination. Many of us take a shower before sex, because, well, we like to be clean before we do the dirty. So why not use that shower as an

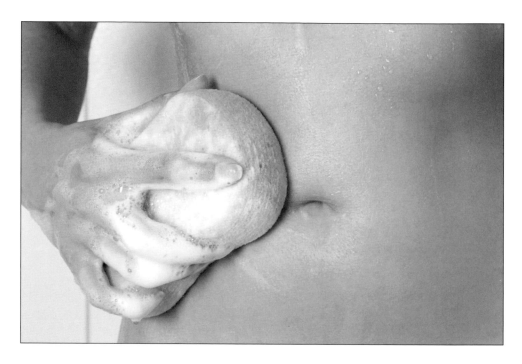

opportunity to get the engines revving before the big event? If you shower alone, and are female, the shower head can be best your best friend, especially if you have a detachable hose. Find the temperature and pressure that works for you, then use the showerhead to your advantage. Water can heighten your senses if you allow it, and you can direct the head to any part of your body you wish.

If you shower with your partner, try washing their hair, soaping them up, and then rinsing them off with the shower head. Spend more time on the sensitive areas of their body. Then reverse the operation. I'm willing to bet by the time it comes to stepping out of the shower, you are both raring to go.

Hack: Give Yourself Permission to Be Naughty

A fun sex life is all about letting loose, living sexy, and learning how to have fun. This hack comes from Bobbie Morgan, editor-in-chief of *A Good Woman's Dirty Mind* (agoodwomansdirtymind.com).

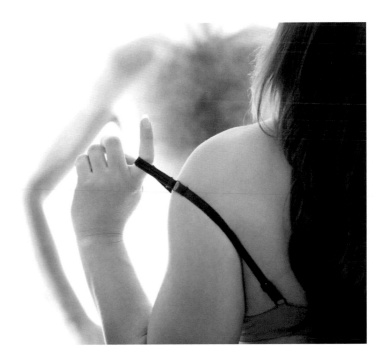

A former lover of my partner described him as a guy who looked like Mister Rogers, with a soul of Dennis the Menace. Being a grownup when it comes to work, raising kids, and taking care of a home is a good thing, but remember that thrill you had as a kid doing something that was wrong, and the excitement you had from pulling it off? A fun sex life is all about breaking the rules and giving yourself permission to be naughty.

Cop a feel at a restaurant, bar, or party—even a family party—when you're sure no one's looking. Slip off to a secluded place like a closet or a bedroom where the risk of being discovered is relatively safe and remotely possible. Scope out a place where you can discreetly pull off having semi-public sex, like behind some trees and bushes, on a balcony, or in a stairwell. Pulling off a small article of clothing like a pair of panties and handing them to your lover in public place is one of the oldest tricks in the book, but it works. So does telling your lover what you're wearing or not wearing under your clothes.

Hack: Create a Sexy Adult Slip-and-Slide

We often think of sex as something that involves only our genitals, but the best sex involves our entire bodies. We are covered in nerves and hidden erogenous zones, many of which are unique and just waiting for your partner to discover. This hack comes from sex blogger Symone "Kitty" Nelson (www.symonekittynelson.com).

Nuru massage is a long-used Japanese style of massage that emphasizes intimacy and the erotic power of touch. Nuru massages are done with both partners fully nude, using a highly slippery gel specially manufactured for Nuru massages. The gel is activated by body heat, which is why nudity is ideal (and the most fun). Apply the gel liberally because the more you apply, the easier it is to glide across your partner's body. I like to compare Nuru to the X-rated, adult version of the slip and slide. Once your area is set up for the massage and you and your partner are on a non-absorbent material, such as large plastic sheet, the fun begins! Use your body to tease and tantalize your partner by rubbing, writhing, sliding, and grinding yourself up against them.

The general rule of Nuru massages has been to use soft-tissue areas such as the breasts and buttocks against hard tissue areas such as the back and vice versa, but do whatever makes you feel sexy and sensual. Start the massages with your partner on their stomach to get them worked up, and then turn them on their back to heat things up even more. Massage in general is a sensual and stimulating way to enhance foreplay and to awaken the senses. Nuru takes that to a whole new level. Where traditional massages focus on hand-to-body stimulation, Nuru emphasizes the use of the entire body. If you want to make your Nuru massage more exciting, you can try taking away one or more of your partner's senses. Blindfolds take away the ability to see and create anticipation, while restraints take away your partner's ability to touch you back, giving you complete control over their body.

Hack: Set Yourself Up for a Sex Dream

Have you ever woken up from a super-sexy dream you just wanted to dive right back into? Dreams can often feel like the real thing, and they're a great place to play out fantasies and get yourself worked up for a real-life partner. In fact, it's even possible for some people to orgasm in their dreams. So how can you enjoy a little sexy time while you're sleeping? Masturbating, reading erotica, or watching pornography right before sleep can help set the tone. A study published in the journal *Dreaming,* in September 2012, also found that those who sleep on their stomachs are more likely to enjoy sexy slumber.

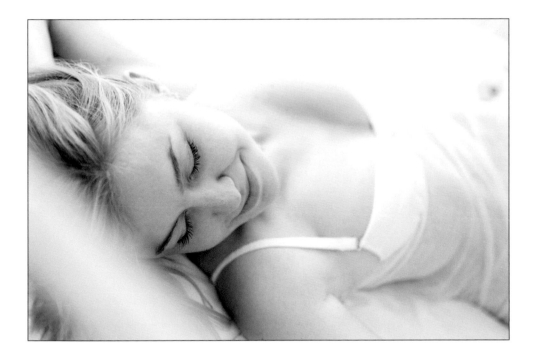

3. In-the-Sack Hacks

Now is when the real fun begins. Once you get the action going, where to take it from there? They say the road to mediocre sex is paved with repetition. So, unless "mediocre" is the kind of sex you want, it's time to mix things up and try something new. That doesn't necessarily mean you have to assemble a sex toy arsenal or muscle your way into acrobatic sex positions. In fact, many of the best sex hacks are so much simpler. They involve making things go more smoothly, avoiding the awkwardness, and getting the position *just* right. In other words, our in-the-sack hacks are about logistics. You become

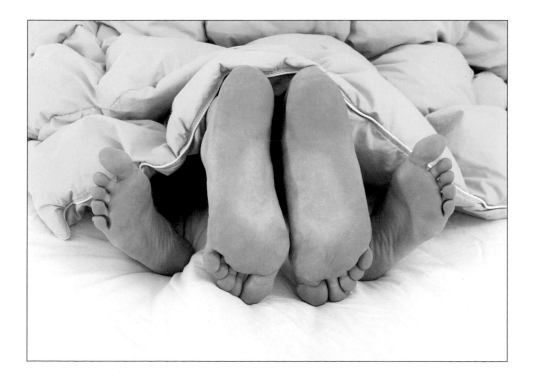

the sexual resource manager, doling out just the right amount of pleasure (or pain) at precisely the right moment. Expect amazing results.

Hack: Know Your Anatomy (and Your Partner's)

This seems too simple. You know anatomy, right? Penis, vagina, clitoris, testicles, done. *Oy.* Sexual anatomy is actually beautifully complex. We have so many different erogenous zones and genital hotspots, but many of us just barely know the basics. After all, this isn't info you ever get in sex-ed. If you want to give and receive great sex, you need to know your partner's basic anatomy—and your own. Pick up a few good sexual references (with pictures!), and then dig in and do your research. Also note that each person's body has its own wonderfully individual quirks. Get the basics down, then apply them to your partner's unique body and desires.

Hack: Become a Scientist of Sex

The best, most satisfying sex often happens as a result of experimentation. The problem is that experimentation can be scary. It means putting ourselves in situations we've never tried before—and situations that may not get us off (boo!). So, the key to getting curious and creative in the bedroom is all about adjusting your expectations and being prepared to fail. Rather than going in with the goal of "succeeding" at something new, head in like a mad scientist looking to try new things—and learn from them. This takes away the pressure of performing and allows you and your partner to experiment and learn about what works best. Failure is a natural part of experimentation—but so is fun!

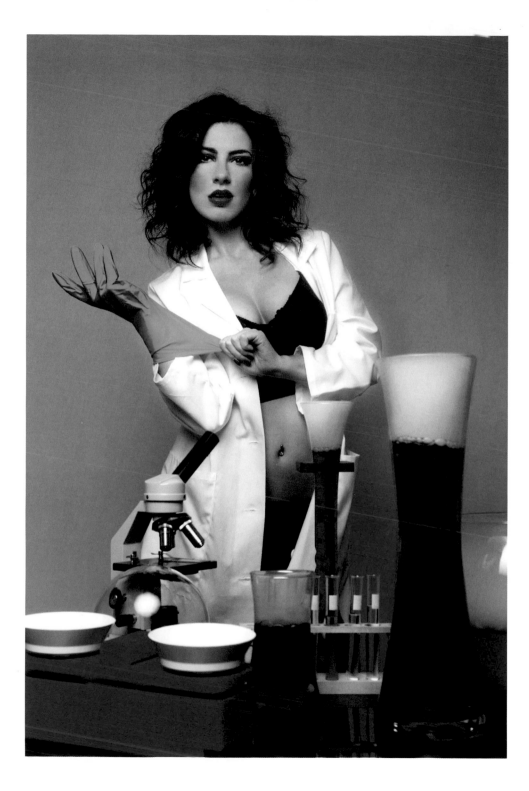

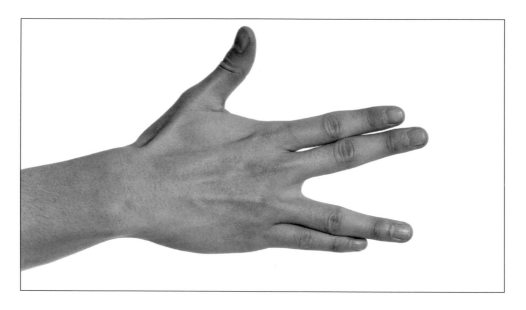

Hack: Giver Her the Vulcan Salute

If you aren't a *Star Trek* fan, or "Trekkie," you may never have heard of the Vulcan Salute, but if you're a man with a female partner, now's the time to get intimate with this hand gesture. Simply flatten your palm, and fully extend and spread your fingers and thumb. Then, bring your pointer and middle fingers together and your little and ring fingers together, leaving a space between your middle and ring finger. Use this gesture to take missionary to a whole new level; make this sign with your hands and put the two fingers on either side of your penis, allowing your partner to grind against your knuckles during intercourse. This hand position provides more friction for the clitoris, which helps many women reach orgasm. The hand gesture means "live long and prosper." Get this one right and you can apply that code to your sex life too!

Hack: Cross Your Legs and Squeeeeze!

Many women feel the need to squeeze their legs together as they approach orgasm. This natural impulse is worth giving in to. You can even intensify

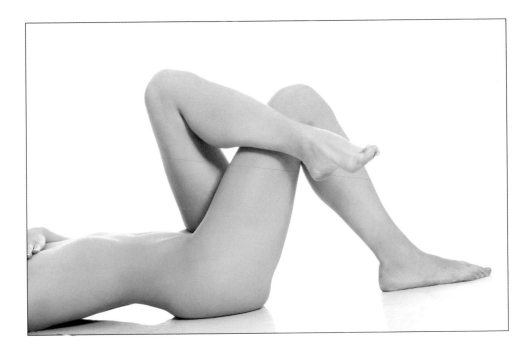

it in some positions by crossing your legs and squeezing even harder. This helps awaken the core muscles involved in orgasm, thus intensifying the sensation. Plus, if you're having penetrative sex, your partner will be able to enjoy the snug fit and additional friction you're creating with your body.

Hack: Install a Lube Dispenser by the Bed

If there's one tip you'll hear from just about every sex geek out there, it's this: use lube. Lots of it. You can never get too much. It makes sex easier. It makes sex more comfortable. Heck, a little extra lubrication even makes condoms more effective because they're less likely to break. Do we have your attention? Check out this hack from one of the Web's top sex toy reviewers, Epiphora (heyepiphora.com).

*Potentially the greatest thing to happen to my sex life since lube itself is my **motion-activated lube dispenser.** Oh, it's marketed as a humble soap dispenser,* *but the potential for perversion is too great. During masturbation and sex is exactly the time when I don't have two free hands with which to acquire lube.*

My lube dispenser set me back forty dollars and holds an impressive eight ounces of fluid. I suggest a medium consistency, water-based lube that won't slide off your sex toy the moment it dispenses. Avoid a lube so thick that it won't move freely through the dispenser. You can adjust how much liquid is dispensed each time, but you'll likely want the default setting. The dispenser is pretty quick to respond when something is thrust under it, so be prepared! It also emits an adorable "bzzzt" sound as it dispenses.

If you're careful, nary a drip will hit the nightstand. But it's true that accidents can happen, and for that, I recommend placing a small tray under the dispenser to catch any spilled lube. The only other downside to this hack is that you may end up using more lube than necessary just because it's fun. Which is not a downside at all.

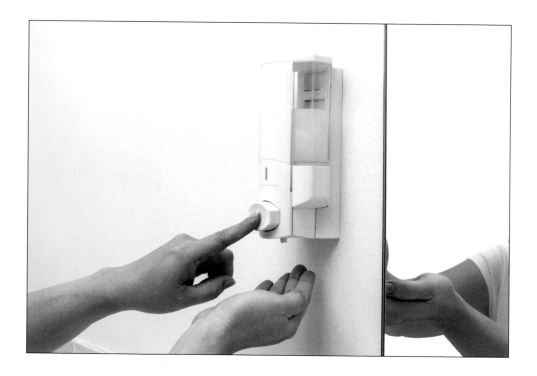

Hack: Get Into Outercourse

Outercourse refers to sex without penetration. This is something you may have experimented with long before you had bid adieu to your virginity, but it can go way beyond the sexually frustrating, pubescent foreplay many people associate with it. Start by rubbing up against your partner when you're spooning in front of the TV, or even at the back of a crowded party. The friction's fun, but getting grabby can also help you and a long-term partner reconnect with the passion you had when you first met. After a good, clothing-optional tussle, you can even take it all the way with erotic massage, mutual masturbation, or mammary intercourse. Just start rubbing up against each other and allow the fun to unfold!

Hack: Use a Desensitizing Lube to Help You Last Longer

The penis wasn't really designed with endurance in mind; research suggests the average time it takes to go from arousal to ejaculation is a mere five to ten minutes. Now, if a quick romp pleases you and your partner, there's nothing to worry about. If it doesn't, a little more longevity may be in order. So, how to last a little longer? One simple way to do that is to try applying a desensitizing lube to the penis. This helps reduce the sensation to the penis and increases the time to orgasm. Just remember that your partner will feel the effects of this stuff too, so it might be best to put some inside a condom.

Hack: Put an Unbalanced Load in the Washing Machine

The washing machine provides just the thing many women crave. No, not fresh, clean laundry—we're talking vibration, and *lots* of it. So, while hopping up on the washing machine and doing your thing during the spin cycle is a well-known trick, try it with a heavy, unbalanced load. Place towels or other heavy laundry on one side of the drum, then fire it up. Your washing machine will be kicking and bucking as much as you and your partner.

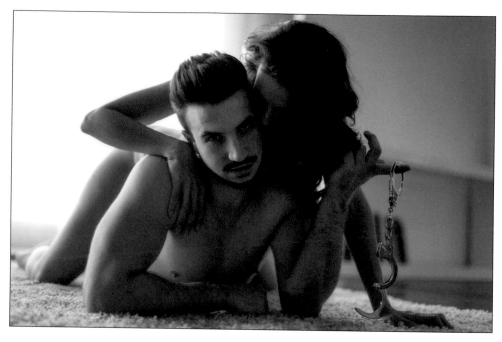

Hack: Switch Roles

If you have a regular sexual partner, you probably follow a pretty standard routine. Next time, instead of the same-old-same-old, try switching roles. If you're usually in charge and get things started, allow your partner take control instead. Switching things up can totally change the sexual dynamic and energy, making sex with a long-term partner feel brand-new—and hotter than ever.

Hack: Play "Everything But"

It's easy to get caught up in getting to intercourse, particularly for heterosexual couples, but there are a lot of other fun and satisfying things to do in bed—and they don't just have to be foreplay. Try playing a game called "Everything But," where the goal is to get your partner off in a new way *that doesn't involve intercourse*. This is a great way to get creative and explore new things with your partner. After all, creativity is what building a beautiful, satisfying sex life is all about.

Hack: Use a Silicone or Oil-Based Lube to Silence a Squeaky Bed Frame

A squeaky bed frame is a minor but cumulative annoyance for sexually adventurous people. But if your neighbors are complaining—or your kids are banging on the door to see what's going on in there—it can really put a damper on an active love life. So how can you keep your bed from announcing your nocturnal habits? Easy: Apply a little silicone or oil-based lubricant to the adjoining parts of the bed. Sure, you could use WD-40, but lube tends to smell a whole lot better. Plus, it's handy!

Hack: Seize the Moment—Any Moment—For Sex

If you have a busy life and long-term relationship—and especially if you have kids—squeezing it in (so to speak) can be really difficult. How to make

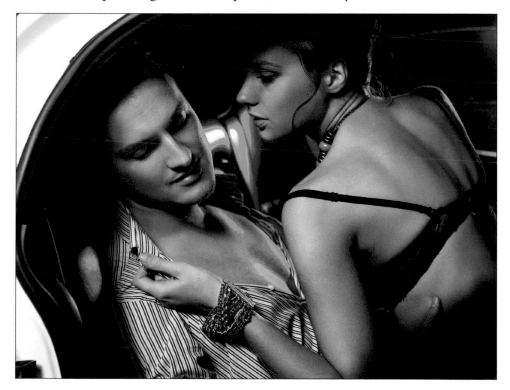

it work? *Just do it*. Do you have a few minutes alone? Go for it. Sometimes, sex is about making sure you don't forget how to do it. Sometimes, even rushed sex in an uncomfortable position is pretty darned good.

Hack: Go Hands Free

Sex is often all about getting a little handsy. Touching, fondling, fingering . . . oh my! For something a little different, try going hands-free. This will force you and your partner to experiment with your noses, mouths, teeth—even your toes—in ways you'd never imagined. Not being able to fast-track your foreplay will also help you explore each other's bodies in new ways—and extend the fun. Plus, you'll probably get hot just thinking about what you *could* do if your hands were an option.

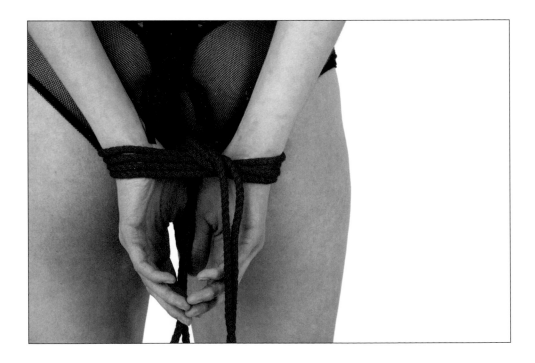

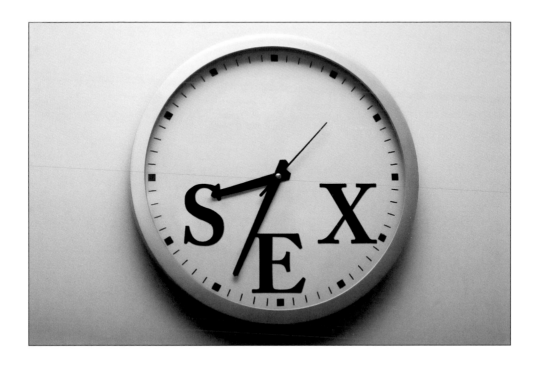

Hack: Rejigger Your Carnal Clock

According to the Great American Sex Survey conducted by sex toy retailer Adam & Eve, sex most often occurs late at night. The problem is that if you're always trying to squeeze your sex life into the last part of your day, you're much more likely to pass out without getting any. Try ditching the notion that sex is a bedtime ritual and look for little openings where you might be able to fit in a fling. Whenever you and your partner have some time to yourselves will do; the most sexually satisfied couples are those who've learned to never discriminate.

Hack: Get Your Room to Just the Right Temperature for Sex

We're often led to believe that the best, wildest, most throw-off-the-reins sex happens in uncomfortable places: the back seat of a car, an elevator, the beach. That can be great fun, but our most sexually experienced friends tell us that the best sex happens when both partners are as comfortable as possible. This hack from top sex toy reviewer Epiphora (heyepiphora.com) is aimed at creating the most optimal environment for great sex—in any season.

During times of the year when temperatures rise or drop insufferably, it can be hard to muster the desire to have sex. To make sex more appealing during these times, I recommend creating the optimum environment for comfortable sex. Don't be afraid to do things that might seem weird. Comfort is all that matters!

For instance, during winter I use a small space heater in the bedroom whenever I have sex. I can set it at the temperature of my choice, and it will heat the room perfectly. This way, we don't have to bury ourselves under the covers. If I remember to turn the heater on early, I can prepare the room in advance, and eliminate shivering altogether. Sometimes, if I set the heater near the end of the bed, my partner and I can even remove our socks during sex!

In the summer, there are a number of things you can do. Fill a spray bottle with cold water, and give yourself or your partner a spritz if you get too hot. Add a fan to the equation and you'll have some nice airflow. Take a cold shower before sex—or after. Have sex in a half-filled inflatable pool! OK. You get the idea.

Hack: Use Yoga Props to Stretch Out Your Session

A yoga teacher will tell you that yoga props, like blocks or straps, improve "posture" and "alignment." Our experts tell us they're good for sex too; whether you're doing downward-facing dog or going at it doggie style, the more comfortable you are, the longer you'll be able to hold the position. This sex hack comes from dating coach and sex educator Rebecca Hiles (friskyfairy.com). Your yoga teacher will totally approve.

I love kneeling for oral and other sex positions, and I love the spontaneity of having sex in places that aren't a bed. Unfortunately, because I'm a bigger person, I find that not only do my hands and knees start to hurt after some time, but occasionally I'll experience my foot or fingers falling asleep if I'm the position for too long. If I'm on a harder surface like a floor or a shower, using an inexpensive yoga mat can help alleviate some of the discomfort. I also find that other yoga equipment can be multifunctional too! Yoga blocks can help lift you up if you and your partner are mismatched in height. A yoga strap is great for helping you pull your legs back over your head, or even simply holding in a position that you enjoy. If you are a larger person, or you have any restrictions on the positions you can do for whatever reason, picking up a yoga mat, a block (or two!), and a strap is awesome. Even if you can move into a number of positions, pick up some yoga basics and an acrobatic position book, and try something new!

4. Oral Sex Hacks

Cunnilingus. Fellatio. Going down. Giving head. Bikini burger. Slurping the gherkin. Call it what you like, but don't underestimate its power. Oral sex isn't just an amazing foreplay technique, it's also an extremely intimate and arousing way to interact with your partner's body all on its own. But if you want to ensure that it's pleasurable for everyone involved (and of course you do, right?), you'll need to follow a few rules. Here are some tips, tricks, and traps to avoid that'll ensure that going down is always a real treat for both of you.

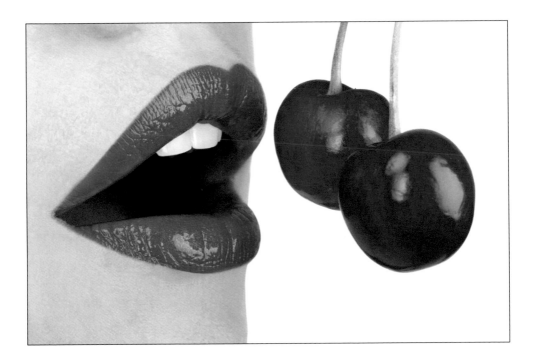

Hack: Improve Oral Endurance by Releasing Neck and Jaw Tension

The biggest complaint most people have about giving oral sex is that it can be really hard work, and sometimes the tension in your neck, jaw, and back forces you to bail before you get the job done. Oral sex can be really athletic—at least for the face and neck—so start by treating yourself like an athlete. First, have your partner gently massage your face, neck, and jaw. This can help get you warmed up and can help release the tension from these areas. (It's also great foreplay!) Then, once you go down, remember to relax, breathe, and let go of tension. Not only will this help improve your endurance, but your partner will be able to sense that you aren't frantically trying to finish things up before your face falls off, which can really kill the sensual mood.

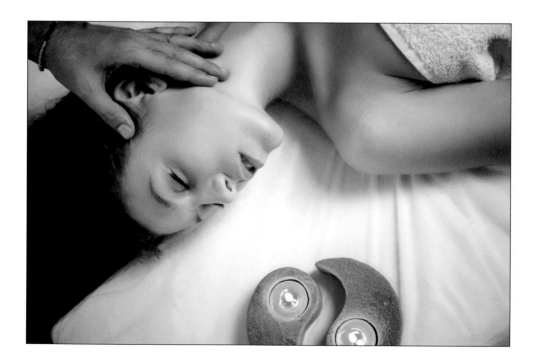

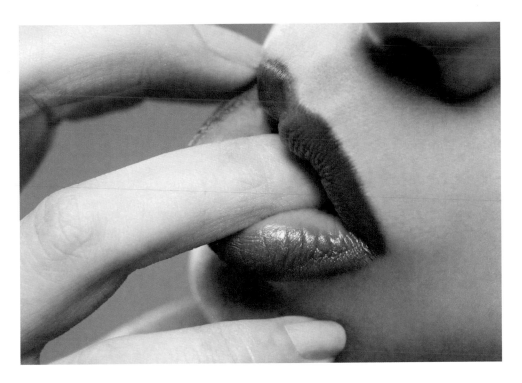

Hack: Fire Up Your Lover by Fellating Their Fingers

The best oral lovers move oh-so-slowly, building tension as they go. One way to do this is to fellate your partner's fingers. Kiss, nibble, lick, and suck those long, lovely appendages, applying some of your favorite oral sex techniques. The fingers have many nerve endings, making this a great sensual teaser. It will also keep your partner's mind on what's to come.

Hack: Save Your Jaw by Varying Your Technique

Want to wow your partner with your oral skills, without getting a case of lock-jaw? This handy sex hack from Mandi at *EROcentric* (erocentric.word-press.com) is a two-for-one special.

At some point or another, most all of us have had a particularly lengthy oral sex session that has ended with a tired and sore jaw. It may have even been severe enough that it ended the session prematurely. Depending on your medical diagnoses (particularly temporomandibular joint disorders) and your physical abilities, there's one simple tip that may help you manage, or even prevent, jaw pain during the act of oral sex.

Variety.

By making sure that your mouth is not open for long periods of time, you can prolong your comfort during oral sex. If you feel your jaw starting to get tired, switch things up by trying new oral sex techniques or by expanding your focus to include other erogenous zones. Lightly kissing your partner's genitals or nibbling on your partner's thighs can provide you with a much-needed break while keeping your partner hot and heavy. If you are still experiencing discomfort, let your mouth rest and focus on intimate touching for a while instead.

By embracing this variety, not only will you end your next oral sex session without a sore jaw, but you'll blow your partner away with your sexual teasing.

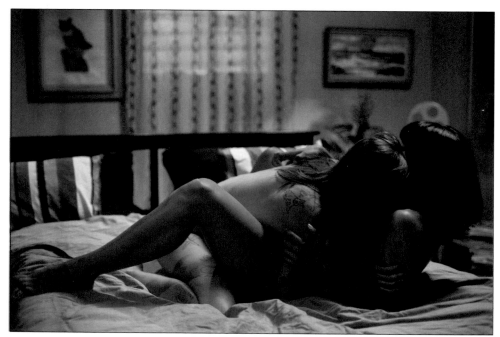

Source: CrashPadSeries.com.

Hack: Get Aroused to Improve Your Ability to "Deep Throat"

We often think of oral sex as a way to arouse our partners, but if you're fellating a penis in particular, it's very important to arouse yourself first. Arousal—and the feel-good hormones that come with it—help open up and relax the throat. This will make giving oral sex more pleasurable for you and for the lucky recipient of your oral energies. Adequate arousal can even make the highly coveted act of "deep throating" possible for some people. After all, arousal is known to relax and open the body, your mouth and throat are no exception.

Hack: Add a Vibrator

To pack a bigger punch with your oral play, consider adding a vibrator. Whether you're pleasing a penis or charming a vulva with your oral skills, press a powerful vibrator against the side of your cheek. Your partner will

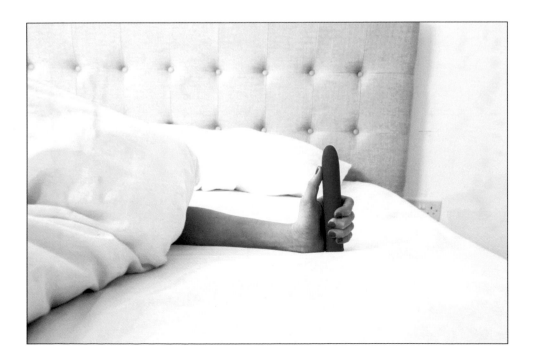

be able to feel the reverberations through your mouth as you suck and lick away, adding a new dimension of sensation.

Hack: Use Heat to Enhance Sensation

Sex is all about sensation. The more variety you can create, the more you'll be able to maintain an element of spontaneity and surprise in your sex life. One thing the genitals really respond to is heat. Next time you're giving oral sex, take a drink of hot water before going down. Then, place your mouth over your partner's penis or vulva, using your tongue to gently stimulate the area in the way your partner prefers. The extra heat will leave you both feverish with desire.

Hack: Create a Cool Tingle by Refrigerating Your Favorite Lube

Using a favorite flavored lubricant can add a new dimension to oral sex, but you can also use lube to add a little temperature play to the mix. Pop a bottle of your favorite lube into the fridge for a few hours, then transfer the cool tingle to your partner through your mouth. This is a great trick for cooling off on hot summer days!

Hack: Clench Your Fist to Stop Your Gag Reflex

A strong gag reflex can really put a damper on giving great oral sex. This popular dentist's trick can help: simply make a fist with a thumb on the inside of the fist and squeeze gently. No one's sure why it works, but whether it has to do with the nerves in your hand, or it just acts as a distraction, it works! This technique is even used to help calm athletes during stressful competitions. As it turns out, it's great for non-athletes playing with a different set of balls as well.

Hack: Follow Your Nose to Additional Stimulation

The key to really pleasing the vulva and clitoris is as plain as the nose on your face. Really. It's easy to get focused on using your mouth, tongue, and lips to please all those glorious folds, but the nose is a smooth, strong digit that can provide a great source of additional stimulation. Try rubbing your nose around the clitoris and along the labia. This spongy piece of cartilage can become the perfect sex toy.

Hack: Train Your Tongue

Your tongue has eight super-strong, ultra-dexterous muscles, making it a powerhouse when it comes to pleasing a partner. Chances are, your tongue can create a lot more sensations than you can even imagine. So, get creative and start thinking about all the things your tongue can do. You could flatten your tongue and lick your partner like a delicious ice cream cone, or make the end of your tongue firm and pointy, flicking it side to side over your lover's sensitive areas. The key is to try all the different strokes and touches you can think of, and see how your partner reacts. If you take the time to

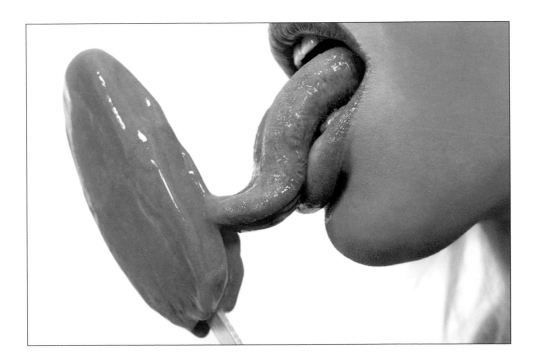

experiment on each other, you'll be able to come up with the moves to (literally) blow each other away.

Hack: Crown Your Love a Pillow Princess

Forget standing on your head. Sometimes, the best orgasms come to those who get nice and comfy. If you're looking to please a female partner with your oral skills, try this hack from professional sex, intimacy, and relationship coach Marla Renee Stewart (marlareneestewart.com).

If you're having sex in the bedroom and are ready to go down on your girl, you want your princess (or queen) to be as comfortable as possible—the more relaxed she is, the better she will be able to achieve an awesome orgasm. Place a pillow or two underneath her butt to lift her pelvis toward your mouth. Not only will she be able to relax more and enjoy the pleasure that you're giving her, but it will help keep your neck from being too strained, especially if she wants you to be there for a while.

Hack: Make Your Partner Feel Delicious

Sex isn't just about anatomy, it's also about psychology. If you really want to get a partner hot and bothered, you have to appeal to both mind and body. This hack comes from porn star and director Cyd St. Vincent.

Who doesn't like a blowjob? Plenty of people don't enjoy them when they are done without any passion. Wanna up your game? The trick to giving great head starts way before your mouth is touching someone's junk.

First, make clear what you are going to do. A little hair pulling make-out while you rub your hand down their torso to make them squirm.

Once you are on your knees, or lying on top, tease them over their underwear. The feeling of a mouth against fabric is the exact thing to get people straining for the next step. This is also when you can get kinda rough—rubbing your teeth over those tighty-whities—whatever it takes to make them feel like you're about to devour them alive.

If you haven't already been talking dirty, now's the time to start running your mouth. Tell them how excited you are.

It's almost time for the main event, but first, pull their underwear to the side. All this build up will make your lover so goddamn hot. They will also feel super good about their body. This is the real hack—making your partner feel like their body is super delicious by having them see and hear how much you enjoy it.

Hack: Eat Pineapple for Better Taste Below the Waist

You might love giving and receiving oral sex, but let's be honest: genitals don't exactly taste like candy. While a partner who's attracted to you is more likely to dig your personal flavor, keeping things fresh down there is kind of like dabbing on some perfume: it isn't necessary, but it's a nice gesture. Pineapples, as well as citrus fruits like oranges or grapefruit, help to balance the vagina's pH, adding a bit of sweetness to its secretions. Eating acidic fruit like pineapple can also make semen taste sweeter. No one's crotch will ever taste like a cupcake, but it's always nice to put in a little extra effort to please your partner and, by extension, yourself!

Hack: Create a Buzzing Sensation With Your Lips

Oral sex is all about creating unique sensations, and the more the better. One really simple technique that can send your partner soaring is to buzz your lips around your partner's clitoris or head of the penis. Start by relaxing your lips and jaw, taking a deep, full breath, and then letting your lips buzz as you exhale. This technique might take a little practice, but it's worth the effort; turning your mouth into a vibrator is sure to surprise your partner and send tingles up his or her spine.

Hack: Get a Cushioned, Non-Slip Mat for Your Shower

The shower is a great place to give and receive oral sex. It's warm, it's wet, and you're both buck naked and squeaky clean. The problem is that most standard showers are pretty small and slippery, which doesn't leave much room for performing your oral gymnastics routine comfortably—or safely. Put down a non-slip mat to avoid slips and falls. A cushioned one will provide the comfort you need to get down on your knees as well.

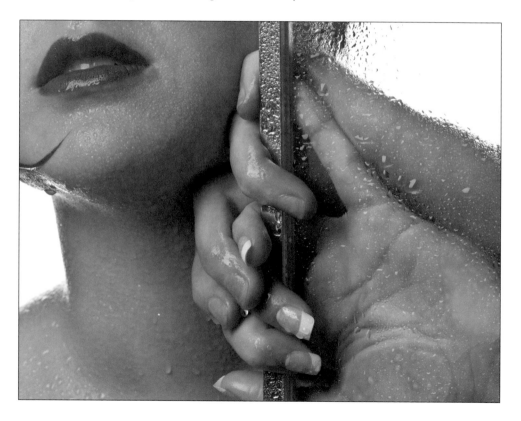

5. Anal Sex Hacks

Once viewed as strictly taboo, in recent years interest in and acceptance of anal sex among young women has been growing. According to the most recent National Survey of Sexual Health and Behavior completed in 2010, 21 percent of American women aged twenty to twenty-nine reported having tried anal sex in the past year. The figure was the same for women aged thirty to thirty-nine. That's a huge increase over earlier research collected by the University of Chicago in 1988 under the National Health and Social Life Survey, which found that about 12 percent of American women aged twenty to twenty-nine had experienced back door action.

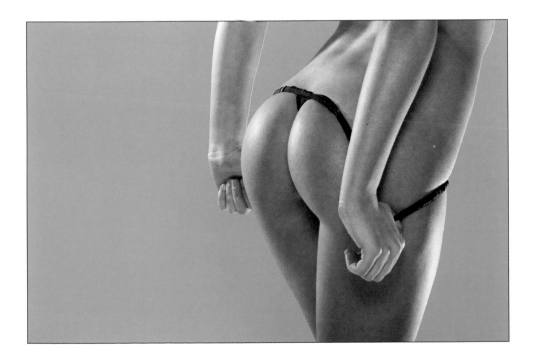

Whether you've tried it or not, what those in the know will tell you is that anal sex can be amazing—and orgasmic. That because the anus is packed with nerve endings and blood vessels. Its proximity to the vagina in women and the prostate in men also means that it provides a new angle for stimulating those sexual organs. So, who can blame people for wanting to tap into that stimulation? After all, variety is the spice of life! As the negative social barriers that have long prevented curious people from trying anal sex begin to fall away, all that's left is a lack of knowledge around anal sex and how to make it safe and pleasurable for those involved. So, a few key points about safety.

First, lubricant is essential. Lots of it. Unlike the vagina, the anus is not self-lubricating. That means that going in without lube can create friction, which can mean pain and even anal tearing. Most anal aficionados recommend either a silicone or oil-based lubricant for your anal endeavors. Choose what works for you.

Next up, toys. They're a great way to test out anal stimulation and they come in a variety of shapes and sizes. There's one thing all anal toys have in common, though: they have a flared base. This prevents the toy from "getting lost." Getting it found again typically involves an emergency room visit, so choose your toys carefully.

Finally, take it slow. Whether you're playing on your own or with a partner, listen to your body's cues, move slowly, relax, and remember that anal sex should not be painful. If you're feeling pain, it might be time to back off a bit and try again. Anal sex can be extremely pleasurable, but only if you play safe. Please do. It's your butt on the line.

Now for the fun part. Here are a few hacks that'll help you give anal a try—and ensure that you enjoy it.

Hack: Stimulate the Prostate Without Penetration

You've probably heard of the hallowed G-spot, the pleasure-packed area found on the front wall of the vagina, but what about the P-spot, or prostate? It's the male equivalent of a G-spot, and the pleasure it can produce is no secret. Because the prostate produces most of the fluid that makes up ejaculate, stimulating it in just the right way can produce longer, deeper orgasms for many people. The walnut-sized gland is found between the bladder and the penis, which means that massaging it often involves anal penetration—but it doesn't have to. This tip for external prostate play comes from porn producer and Crash Pad Series star Nikki Silver.

I recently learned that one can stimulate the prostate from the outside of the body. How to do it? Press on the area between the balls and the anus. Try to move your fingers down and back, toward the tailbone. You will begin to feel a soft, but firm, spot. This is the prostate gland. You'll have to experiment on what feels good for your partner, but try making a gentle, upward scoop motion with lube on your hand in conjunction with stroking the cock.

Hack: Put a Condom On It for Safer, Cleaner Fun

Condoms make for safe sex, and not just when you put them on a penis. In fact, when it comes to anal sex, wrapping up anything that is inserted into the anus is a smart move. While the butt may be a pleasure palace, it's also home to its own bacterial ecosystem, one that is not a friend to the vagina or mouth. Covering up with a condom can help ensure that sex toys stay sterilized for later use, and that a penis that's taken the back entry can still go through the front door.

Hack: Eat More Fiber

A healthy diet is important for a healthy sex life, but it's especially important for healthy, pleasurable anal sex. The anus isn't a receptacle for feces, but they do pass through on their way out of the body. If things aren't, er, running smoothly, this can lead to irritation and muscle strain, which can make anal play uncomfortable—or even painful. And hey, eating a diet rich

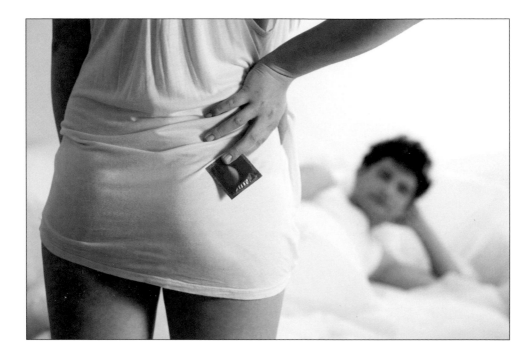

in unprocessed foods, including raw fruits and vegetables, is good for you anyway.

Hack: Use a Powerful Massager to Make Penetration Easier

In order for anal sex to work—and by "work," we mean occur pleasurably rather than painfully—it's important that the anal muscles be relaxed. Clenching can make penetration more difficult, thus spoiling all your butt-centric fun. One way to help relax the area is to use a powerful personal massager or vibrator on the buttocks and around the anal opening to help relax the area and the anal sphincter. This, in itself, can be a real turn-on, but it also helps to make anal penetration easier and more pleasurable. When you move on to penetration, be sure to start slowly, use plenty of lube, and communicate with your partner. Oh, and have fun!

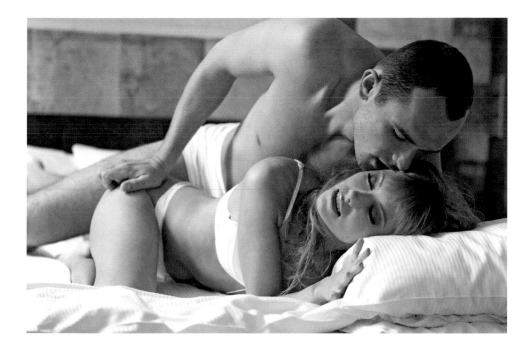

Hack: Come First, Bum Later

For many people, anal play can be as pleasurable—if not more pleasurable—than any other sex act. It is even possible to have an anal orgasm. However, the key to pleasurable anal sex is relaxation and arousal. Sometimes, that's best achieved when anal play comes as a second-course sex act. Try using a tried-and-true method to get off before getting into anal play. Having an orgasm will relax your pelvic floor and make your body—including your butt—less sensitive to pain and more responsive to pleasure.

Hack: Be Open to Trying Again

For many people, anal sex is a new experience. While you never know what you'll like until you give it a try, sometimes it takes more than one taste to develop an affinity for a particular flavor. Anal sex in particular is a very new and different sensation. So, if it doesn't produce fireworks the first time, consider trying again. Plus, the knowledge that the first time might not work out as expected takes the pressure off of you and your partner. You might have an amazing time, you might not. The key is to explore, experiment, and be willing to try again.

6. Sex Talk Hacks

Dirty talk is hardly groundbreaking stuff, but what may surprise you is how much of a difference a little pillow talk can make in your sex life. According to research published in 2013 by Elizabeth Babin, an expert on health communication at Cleveland State University in Ohio, sexual communication and sexual satisfaction are closely linked. The study also found that those who had apprehension about talking about sex were less likely to enjoy it.

Whether you're navigating consent, ensuring that you get what you need, or working to be a better sexual partner, talking dirty is as important as the deed itself. The good news is that sexual communication is a skill, and

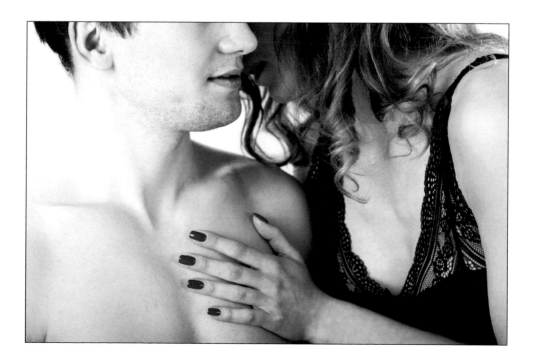

it's one that you can learn and practice over time. Fortunately, we have a few hacks to make your work a whole lot easier—and sexier!

Hack: Practice Aural Sex

Talking about sex is easy for some people, but many others get tongue-tied in trying to express their needs and desires. So how can you ensure that only the sexiest words drip off your tongue in the heat of the moment? Try this tip from Jenne Davis, blogger and head honcho at clitical.com.

When we have sex we should be using all five of our senses, but so often we forget how important our sense of hearing can be. Hearing your partner talk dirty is great, but for some, talking dirty is not an easy thing to do. This is where dirty or erotic stories can come in handy.

Many women report that they enjoy reading erotica. So, by combining your favorite erotic scene into your lovemaking, you can add a new dimension to sex

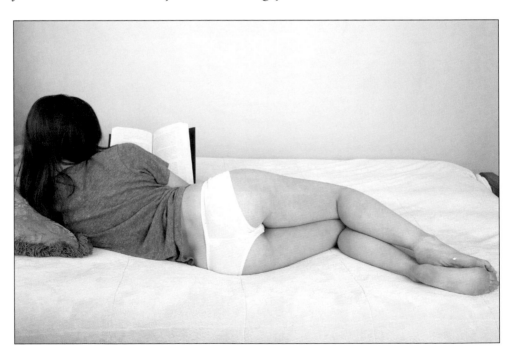

play. First, find a short story that you enjoy. There are plenty of shorts on the net that are free, or you can purchase an anthology of erotica that fits into your particular area of kink or fantasy.

Then, practice reading it out loud when you are on your own. Once you are confident, settle down with your partner and begin to read to them. You can of course take it in turns to read the story; this is your scene and you can do whatever you choose with it!

I'm willing to bet that by the time you've finished reading, both of you are in the mood for some great sex.

Hack: Negotiate a Hook-Up in One Minute Flat

"Hook-up culture" is here to stay, making navigating safe, fulfilling sex with a new partner a game-changing sexual skill. While your fantasies of lassoing that sexy someone may involve little more than smoldering eye contact and the hasty removal of each other's clothes, communication is key to ensuring pleasure for both of you. This sex hack comes from performance artist, actor, and educator Ignacio Rivera (AKA Papi Coxxx).

Words like "negotiation," "safe word," "safer sex," and "boundaries" are said to be necessities in cultivating and maintaining intentional, sex-positive consent culture. I've facilitated extensive workshops on the process one takes to understanding their needs and desires. I've worked with people and created tools for people to express those desires. I've often described this process as a beautiful, lifelong journey to a relationship with yourself and with others. So, how do we do it? How does one pack a lifetime of sexuality trial and error or lessons learned into a lustful encounter that requires you to get down to business, safely?

Before you can work at a successful "Wham Bam Thank You Ma'am/Man," you need to work on you. Having at least an idea of what you want, what makes you hot, or thinking about what you DON'T want is a great start. So let's break it down.

- *Safety:* *What would make this a safer space/safer encounter for you? Is it safe where you have this quickie? Does it have more to do with making sure you have a safe word to stop anything that feels uncomfortable with little to no processing? Is it about safe(r) sex? What does safer sex mean to you? Define these for yourself.*
- *Boundaries*: *You should have had time to think about what some of your top boundaries are. Do your boundaries revolve around what you are willing to do with your body? Are your boundaries around safer sex, sober sex, humiliation, or restrictions on certain words/references to you?*
- *Triggers*: *This word is tossed about and shouldn't be. For me, a trigger is when something happens or is said that puts you into a state of shutting down, brings you to a place of trauma, and could be damaging. Triggers are closely related to boundaries because you can set up boundaries to aid in making sure you are not triggered. In order to do this, you have to be aware of those triggers. Make sense?*
- *Desire*: *What do you want to get out of this tryst? What floats your boat at that moment?*
- *Outcome*: *What is your end goal? Do you want to cum? Do you want tenderness? Do you want aggressiveness? Do you want to be left wanting more? Do you want this to be quick and nasty? Do you want to exchange numbers or be done and walk away?*

The point of a one-minute negotiation hook-up is to go into it knowing (or at least having an idea) of what you want, desire, lust for, and need. Have these bullet points in your head; knowing these things beforehand can make a sprightly sexual encounter that much more satisfying. Remember, you can always reassess and change your mind about anything.

Now go forth and hook up!

Hack: Use Tumblr to Share Ideas with a Partner

Pornography gets a bad rap, but it can actually play a very important role in sexual relationships. It's a great way to come up with new ways to spice up your sex life, get you hot under the collar, and generate a ton of sexual energy between you and your partner. And, if you're a little shy about asking for what you want, sending a dirty picture can be a lot easier—and hotter —than spelling it out. This sex hack comes from JoEllen Notte of *The Redhead Bedhead*, an educator, writer, and consultant on all things sex.

Shy about discussing sex with your partner? Want to try something new in bed but you're not sure how to bring it up? Want to try sexting but don't want your pictures to land on the internet? Tumblr to the rescue!

One of the greatest resources at the hands of the modern fornicator is Tumblr porn—it's like catalog shopping for better sex! The site is full of shareable sexual images. Set up an account with your partner and get ready to revolutionize your sex life. How?

Use it for inspiration. Tumblr is like Pinterest for sex—there's lots of stuff that looks amazing. It may not look anything like the picture when you do it, but you'll have a blast trying.

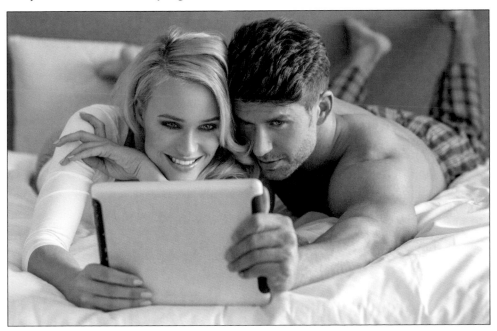

Use it to sext without compromising your own security. No more struggling to get that just-right picture of yourself and then sending it out into the cloud—find a super hot image, reblog it and add the caption: "Tonight, this is us," and it's on! Use it to ask for what you want. Sometimes it's scary to tell a partner you want to try something new. Sometimes it's hard for partners to visualize what that something new is all about. Find a picture of what makes you hot and let them decide if it turns them on too.

Sexual communication can be tricky. Tumblr porn makes it quick, easy, and super hot!

Hack: Tell Your Partner What You'd Like Them to Do Right Now

We hope that all your sexual partners have the best, most orgasmic intentions, but sometimes, they just get things sooo wrong. Unfortunately, telling someone how to do better in the moment can often sound a lot like criticism. And criticism kills boners. Fast. One way to frame this conversation in a positive way is to say, "You know what I'd *really* like you to do to me right now? _____." Then fill in the blank with something that will work for you. This sexy little saying puts the conversation in a positive light and, instead of disempowering your partner, puts them in control of your pleasure. Hot!

Hack: Practice "the Talk" With a Friend Before Trying it on a Partner

Ever struggled with bringing up safe sex with a new partner? This hack from sex educator and writer Ashley Manta (ashleymanta.com) will help you get through the full disclosure—before you take your clothes off.

Since I have genital herpes, I used to jokingly refer to having "the talk" with my prospective partners as "dropping the H-bomb." For me, it is easier to get it out of the way up front—on the first date. (That's not to say it's best for everyone. You need to operate according to your own values and comfort levels.) If you have a positive STI status to disclose, it can be a daunting conversation. These tips can help:

- ***Go in with a plan.*** *Know what you're going to say in advance and make a practice run with a friend if you're nervous.*
- ***Be clear.*** *This is not the time for euphemisms or ambiguity. Give the date of your last STI screening and the results, then break it down into "what does that mean for me" terms.*
- ***Don't take it personally.*** *I've had a myriad of responses to my disclosure, from a casual shrug to someone getting up and leaving. Just remember, this isn't about you. There is a lot of societal stigma surrounding STIs and some people haven't had much or any experience meeting someone who lives with one.*
- ***Leave the door open.*** *Even if the person doesn't have an immediately welcoming reaction, they may just need time to process or do some research.*
- ***Be gentle with yourself.*** *This is hard and you're doing a brave thing. Make time for self care!*

7. Sexual Health Hacks

Sexual health is big deal. Whether it's keeping the physical side of things in check by protecting yourself and your partners from sexually transmitted infections (STIs) and unwanted pregnancies, or navigating sexual dysfunction or gynecological/urinary problems, great sex starts with a healthy, happy body. Actually—scratch that. It gets better: great sex actually helps *contribute* to a healthy, happy body. Sex has been shown to reduce stress, boost mood, lead to better sleep, relieve pain, and even keep you looking and feeling younger. So, even if you take the time to exercise, eat right, and take care of your body, your feel-good formula may still be missing something:

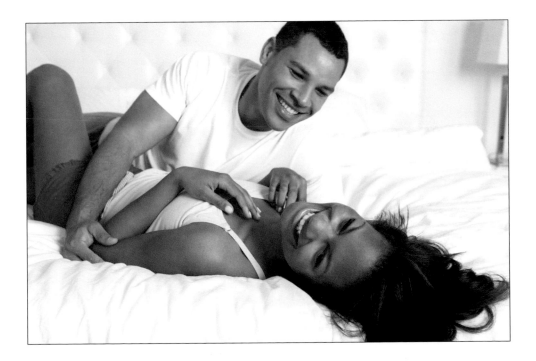

sex! Think of it as your own orgasmic feedback loop. The key is to keep that cycle going. Here are some of our top sexual health hacks to help ensure that your body—and your sex life—is the happiest and healthiest ever.

Hack: Feel Entitled to Pleasure

It doesn't matter if you're a few pounds heavier than you'd like, are sporting a big ol' pimple, or are dealing with other body image issues. If you use your appearance as a guide to feel worthy of sexual pleasure, you are missing out on all the great sex you could be having right now. Enjoying sexual pleasure is a part of being human. It's yours for the taking. So get over your insecurities and seek to enjoy your body's amazing sexual abilities.

Hack: Use a Vibrator to Keep Your Clitoris Humming As You Age

A vibrator can deliver pleasure right now. Wham, bam, thank you battery-operated vibrating device. But a vibrator can also help improve your sexual health, especially when age and inactivity diminish arousal and the strength of your orgasms. This hack from sex writer, educator, and speaker Walker Thornton (walkerthornton.com) is simple: use a vibrator.

Some older women report weaker orgasms over time—using a vibrator can add the necessary extra stimulation to get your clitoris humming. And, if you have a partner, he or she can use the vibrator to supplement other sexual activity. Use a small vibrator during oral sex as well as intercourse, or use sex toys for mutual masturbation. Sexual pleasure does not have to be primarily focused on penetrative sex.

Use sex toys to spark your arousal. It's like practicing anything—once you begin to experience sexual desire and become aroused, it can lead to higher levels of arousal. If you need help getting in the mood, try using a vibrator before sex to get your body and mind engaged and ready. You'll be thinking about sex and your body will already be all warmed up.

Hack: Sync Your Sex Life Up With Your Cycle

Feeling friskier at certain times of the month is all part and parcel of the female reproductive cycle and the monthly hormonal changes that go with it. According to research published in the *Journal of Sexual Medicine* in 2013, there is an ideal time of the month to have an orgasm: day fourteen of the menstrual cycle. Hormonal changes around this time actually cause the clitoris to swell in size by 15 to 20 percent. The clitoral artery also becomes less constricted, allowing for better blood flow. Day fourteen is also around the time when ovulation happens, so it makes sense that the body is gunning for some action. Fourteen isn't a magic number, though; women's cycles tend to vary. If you want to know your sexiest day, listen to your body or consider tracking your cycle. These changes make it easier for you to get turned on, so why not take advantage?

Hack: Build a Safer Sex Arsenal

We all know that safe sex is important, but sometimes it can feel like the least sexy thing *ever*. It can be clinical, fiddly, and can slow down the momentum, but it doesn't have to if you know how to keep safer sex fun and creative. Once you've tried some different products (condoms, lubricant, dental dams, etc.) and have figured out what works for you, stock up on the products that do the best job of keeping you safe without spoiling your fun. Then, build yourself a kit or stock your bedside table with everything you need to play safe. That way, instead of throwing caution to the wind and forgoing safety altogether, you won't have any excuses. Plus, if you stick to the same products, you'll be able to learn how to work those into your sex play in a way that doesn't spoil the mood. Safe sex that's also super fun? Now that's sexy!

Hack: Eat an Apple Every Day to Improve Lubrication

An apple a day has been said to keep the doctor away, but this healthy practice may do a whole lot more. A study published in the Archives of

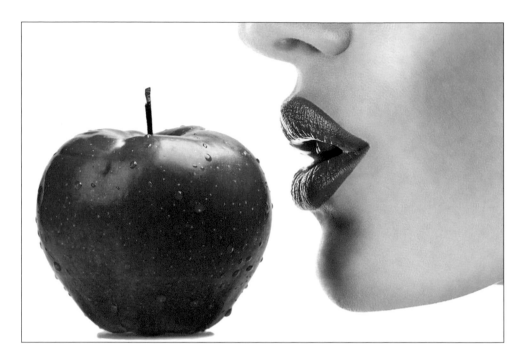

Gynecology and Obstetrics in 2014 suggests that eating more apples may lead to better sex for women. In the study, daily apple consumption was found to increase lubrication and overall sexual function. This effect was attributed to the healthy polyphenols and antioxidants found in apples, which can help improve blood flow and therefore arousal. Apples also contain a common female sex hormone called phloridzin, which plays a major role in vaginal lubrication. So go help yourself to a big, juicy apple. Couldn't hurt, right?

Hack: Use a Condom to Make Your Own Dental Dam

Dental dams. Many people don't use them because they don't think need to or they don't know where to get them. This thin square of latex is placed over the vulva to protect a partner who is performing oral sex. A dental dam is also a good idea when rimming, or orally stimulating the anal area. Dental

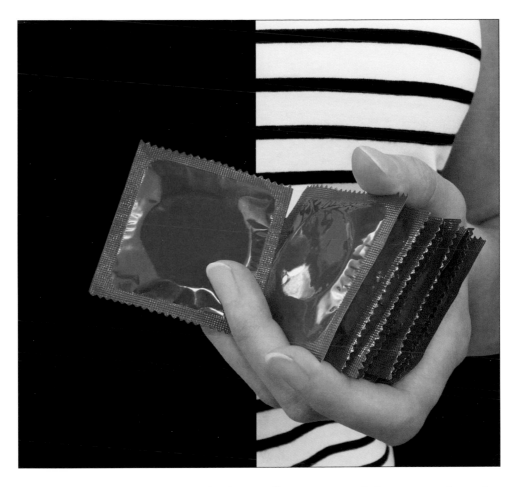

dams help prevent the spread of sexually transmitted diseases and, in the case of anal play, protect your partner from dangerous bacteria. So, yeah, you need one. If you need one in a pinch, you can make your own. Simply cut the tip off a condom, then slice down the length of the remaining tube to create a latex sheet. Voila! Safe oral pleasure waits.

Hack: Learn to Love Your Naked Self

There's nothing sexier than sexual confidence. If you see your body for the strong, sexy thing that it is, your sex life will reflect that. If you hate your

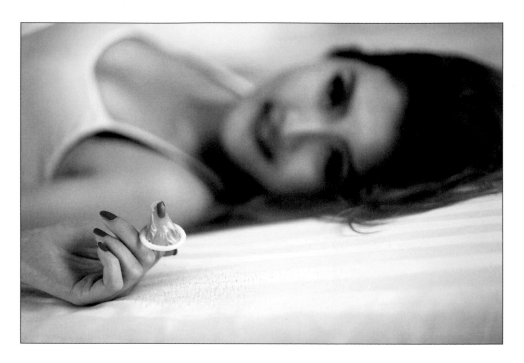

body and spend most of your sexy time worrying about what is or isn't showing or what might be jiggling or what your partner thinks, well, you won't have much time to enjoy yourself or please your partner, will you now? If someone is hot and horny for you, that person thinks you're sexy. Don't second-guess it, own it. Then take that sexy body to the bedroom and show your lover just what it can do.

Hack: Smell Your Sex Toys

Smell your sex toys. Yup, this might sound like a pervy idea, but the smell test is important. Why? Because many sex toys—particularly budget-conscious ones—contain phthalates, a class of chemicals often used to make plastics, inks, paints, industrial lubricants, and adhesives. Many phthalates have been found to have carcinogenic properties and, while they're still used in many plastic products, they're dangerous enough that the government has banned

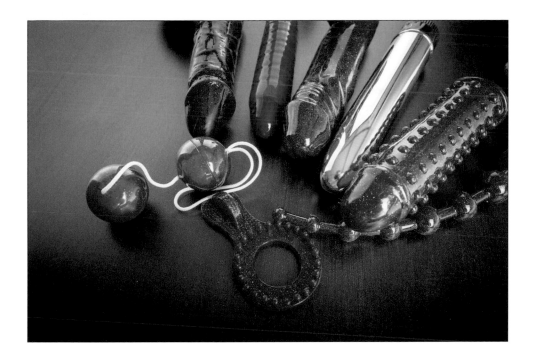

them from being used in baby toys. And yet, there's no law against using them in products you might touch to and insert into your most sensitive areas. Now *that's* gross!

So what can a sex toy's smell tell you? Toys that contain phthalates often have a distinct rubbery, chemical, or "new car" smell. If the toy also has a bendy or squishy texture and is made of jelly-like rubber, vinyl, or PVC, it probably contains phthalates.

So follow your nose—or seek out higher quality toys that are made of stainless steel, medical grade silicone, or glass instead.

Hack: Learn to Get in the Mood

Women in particular often cite a low libido for not getting down and dirty very often. While everyone has a different sex drive, it's important to recognize the difference between not being in the mood and not being able to get in the mood. Rather than just saying "no" when you're really feeling ambivalent, try leaving things a bit more open and allowing for some kissing, foreplay, or cuddle time. Maybe it'll go all the way, maybe it won't. But being open to your partner's advances can help keep the lines of communication open and keep things rolling in the future.

Hack: Leave the Lights On

Sex is a sensual thing. Vision is a sense. Why leave it out? Instead of worrying about how your partner will see you, let your partner look. Not only will you give a good show, but you'll also get to see your partner's reaction. You'll both feel more turned on.

Hack: Share the Glove

When gloves get mentioned in a sexual context, it's almost always in a wrist-snapping, get-ready-for-your-prostate-exam sort of way. But gloves are more than just a racy primetime joke; they're another great way to protect yourself and your partner. This sex hack comes from sex blogger and sex toy reviewer Mandi from *EROcentric* (erocentric.wordpress.com).

Gloves are useful for a variety of reasons and during a variety of activities. First and foremost, they protect both partners from the spread of sexually transmitted infections if there are any cuts or abrasions on one's fingers or hands. During manual stimulation of the vagina or anus, they can be very helpful in creating a smooth surface and preventing small, painful nicks or scrapes that fingernails can cause. When exploring anal stimulation, they can reduce anxiety that some individuals may have about potentially coming into contact with feces by providing a barrier.

When using gloves for sexual purposes, be sure to check with your partner(s) for latex allergies—or stick with non-latex materials (such as vinyl, nitrile, or polyurethane). And next time you're putting together a safe-sex

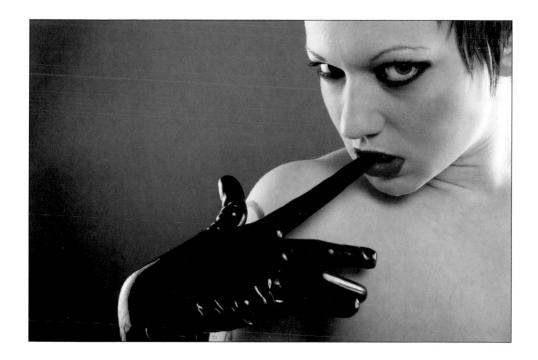

overnight bag, be sure to include a glove or two along with your condoms, dental dams, and lubricant!

Hack: Sleep in the Buff

One of the key indicators of sexual health—and perhaps health in general—is libido. Now, everyone's natural libido is unique, but if you rarely or never feel like having sex, that could signal a problem, if not for your health, then certainly for your relationship. Once you've checked with your doctor to ensure that a health issue isn't interfering with your drive, try sleeping au naturale. According to a survey of 100,000 people conducted by the University of Washington in Seattle, 34 percent of sexually satisfied women and 38 percent of sexually satisfied men always sleep in the buff. Not only does skipping the PJs get you halfway there, but lying skin-to-skin also helps

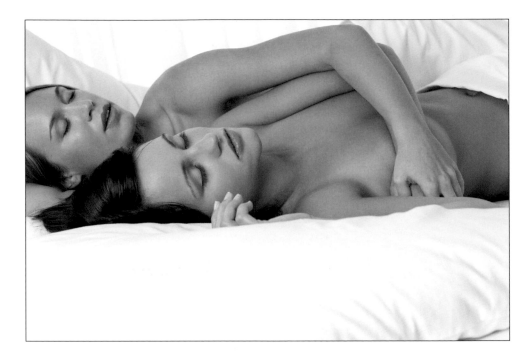

the body secrete the hormones that make you crave your partner. And think about it: Your partner is right there, naked and available. And so are you!

Hack: Drink More Water

Sex might be fun, but it's still exercise. So, if you typically hit the gym with a water bottle in hand, why not do the same before hitting the sack? For women, drinking water helps keep vaginal tissues moist and improves lubrication, making for smoother, better sex. Plus, because the body is mostly made of fluid, keeping those levels topped up should help ensure that everything's working at its best, helping you work toward a great orgasm.

Hack: Vinegar Your Vajayjay

Have you ever tried to do a hard workout when you're under the weather? Didn't go so well, right? The same goes for sex, and while the health of your whole body is key to a great sex life, it also pays to zero in on keeping your privates in tip-top shape; the healthier your naughty bits are, the hotter your sex life has the potential to be. This sexual health hack from professional sex, intimacy, and relationship coach Marla Renee Stuart (marlareneestewart.com) is aimed at keeping hard-working vaginas everywhere ready for action.

Our vaginas tend to fluctuate in terms of the amount of bad and good bacteria that we have. The more acidic foods we take in, the more acidic our vaginas. The vagina is a naturally acidic environment, so alkaline foods are best for balancing the vagina. But sometimes, we don't eat the best foods for us or don't properly check our diet to see if the food we eat is alkaline. Fortunately, you can help keep your vagina looking, feeling, and smelling its best, even when your diet goes off track. The secret? Apple cider vinegar. If your vagina starts to feel off, try diluting some apple cider vinegar and douching with it. This will help get your vagina's pH in balance—and get you ready for your next sexual adventure!

Hack: Practice Yoga

The ancient practice of yoga probably wasn't intended to make you look sexy to onlookers, but hey, when you get flexible enough to get your legs up around your neck, people get certain ideas about your abilities. Actually, they might be on to something. According to a study published in the *Journal of Sexual Medicine* in 2009, regular yoga practice was found to improve several aspects of sexual function in women, including desire, arousal, orgasm, and overall satisfaction. Anecdotally, yoga is also believed to combat erectile dysfunction in men. Yoga also has a great philosophy: it encourages people to focus on the journey, rather than being so goal-oriented. Now there's a tip you can take to the bedroom. Plus, when it comes to getting into more advanced sexual positions, a little extra strength and flexibility is a sex hack of its own.

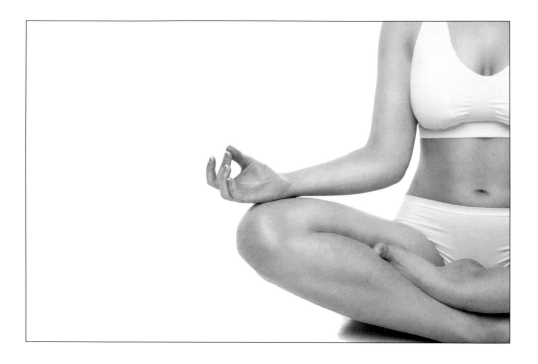

Hack: Use Lube to Turn Back the Clock

Any sexpert worth his or her salt will tell you that you can never have too much lubricant. It's cheap, it's simple, and it reduces the biggest barrier to mind-blowing sex: too much friction. Sex is all about friction, of course, but too much makes things sticky rather than smooth, painful rather than pleasurable. According to Walker Thornton, a writer and sex educator who caters to post-menopausal women, lube can save your sex life. Her hack explains how.

Lube is the best thing you could ever buy for yourself in the sex department. Lubricant is like hand cream for your vulva and clitoris. The hormonal changes of menopause often lead to a decrease in natural lubrication and, with other age-related issues, vulvar and vaginal tissues become irritated and tender to the touch when dry.

The old standby, "just put a little spit on your fingers" routine? Forget it. Invest in a good lube. Think you don't need lubrication? You do. Everything is improved with lubrication. Lube makes fingers, toys, penises, and tongues glide along your most delicate areas. Lubricants help with insertion by reducing friction. A thin layer of lube -–silicone, water- or oil-based, depending on your needs—protects the skin and makes everything feel better. (Remember: Silicone lubes can damage silicone-based sex toys, while oil-based lubes can break down latex condoms, making them more likely to break.) Sensations are enhanced when there's less drag or resistance. You'll find good quality lubricants in sex toy shops, online, or in your local drug store in unscented or scented versions.

Hack: Sleep In to Boost Your Sex Drive

The key to better sex is to spend more time between the sheets—sleeping, that is. According to research published in the *Journal of Sexual Medicine* in 2015, each additional hour of sleep a woman gets increases the likelihood of sex with a partner by 14 percent, which the researchers attribute to an increase in desire. Many busy women feel like they don't have time for sleep *and* sex. Research suggests you should go for the sleep. The sex will take care of itself.

Hack: Use Simple, Natural Coconut Oil as Lube

There are a lot of safe, high-quality sex lubes on the market today. That being said, most of the slippery stuff has its drawbacks. Water-based lube can dry up too fast, and doesn't cut it for anal play. Silicone lube can damage silicone sex toys. Plus, if you're the granola type, you might appreciate keeping things natural around your most sensitive areas. Coconut oil has been hailed as a "super food" with a mile-long list of near-magic properties. And hey, now you can even use it for sex. Its thick texture makes it great for anal sex, its taste and texture make it appealing for oral sex, and it even has anti-fungal and antibacterial qualities. It also makes a great moisturizer and massage cream. Plus, it has a faint coconut smell; it's like having sex at the beach! As

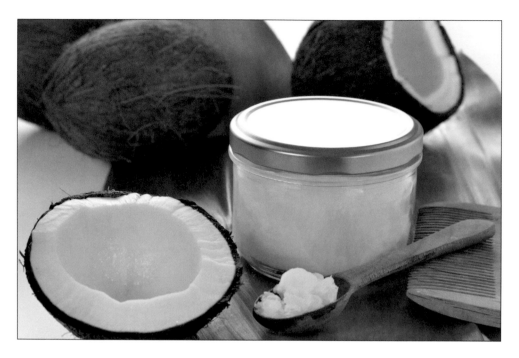

with all oil-based lubricants, however, coconut oil is not compatible with latex condoms.

Hack: Make Your Wine Red

Alcohol is a common social lubricant, but if you're looking to get lucky, it might be best to skip the extra drink and focus on your flirting skills. Too much giggle water can inhibit the parts of the central nervous system that are important for sexual arousal and orgasm. If you are downing a few drinks, though, make them red wine. A study published in the *Journal of Sexual Medicine* in 2009 found that moderate intake of red wine is linked to better sexual health in women. Drinking a glass or two of red wine per day was associated with better sexual desire, lubrication, and overall sexual function compared to non-drinkers and heavy drinkers. Men can reap the benefits here as well. Research published in the *Nutrition Journal* in 2012 found that a compound in red wine could increase levels of testosterone. Cheers!

Hack: Watch Porn

Porn is often criticized as being bad for sex. In fact, research published online in the *Journal of Sexual Medicine* in 2015 suggests that men who watch porn experience more desire for their real-life sexual partners. A survey conducted in 2013 by sex toy manufacturer Ann Summers found that up to 55 percent of women watch porn on their own, while 96 percent reported watching it with a partner, saying it improves sex. As it turns out, watching a few dirty videos isn't just fun for one, it can stoke the fires for playtime with a partner too.

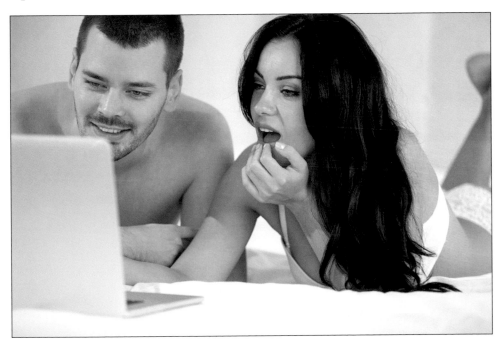

8. High-Tech Sex Hacks

We're all guilty of being a little too in love with our gadgets. If you're like most people, you probably already spend every other minute staring into your smart phone's shiny face, quivering with anticipation for each incoming message or social media update. In fact, when branding expert Martin Lindstrom examined people's brains in an MRI machine to see how they responded to images and sounds from their smart phones, he found that the subjects' brains responded to the sound of their phones the same way they would respond to the presence of a girlfriend, boyfriend, or close family member. In other words, their phones elicited feeling of honest-to-goodness, real love.

In recent years, there has been a massive increase in the ways in which people can connect with each other. There are webcams, sexting, and apps.

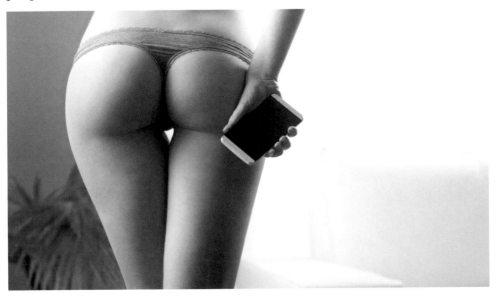

There are remote-controlled vibrators and dildos that can be controlled by a computer program. There are even increasingly realistic sex robots that promise to give the biggest, best orgasm ever.

So, while sex is as old as, well, life itself, is it any wonder that even this most natural of processes is going high tech? Here are some of our top hacks for making sure that your adventures with sex and technology always have a happy ending.

Hack: Create a Phone Sex Toolkit

While sexting is definitely more common and convenient, many people still want to get dirty with a personal touch. And for those who are slogging it out in sexless, long-distance relationships, phone sex can be the best way to keep those fires burning until your next reunion. But just like any kind of sex, satisfying a phone sex partner is an art. This sex hack comes from sex educator, author, and former phone sex operator Ashley Manta (ashleymanta.com).

For the best phone sex experience, it's helpful to have some or all of the following items together:

- *A phone charger. Use a land line if possible (better sound quality), but if not, have your cell phone plugged in to the charger. It's amazing how quickly batteries can drain, especially if you're using a Bluetooth headset (or toy, we'll get there in a sec).*
- *A hands-free headset or Bluetooth headset (having both hands free is incredibly useful).*
- *Something to drink. Your throat will get dry from talking (or moaning!).*
- *Toys and lube. But you might want to consider:*
  - *Whether you want to produce sexy noises—or not. Do you want to use the toy as a sound effect? Pick one that's on the noisy side, like the Magic Wand Original. If you'd prefer a quiet toy that you can use*

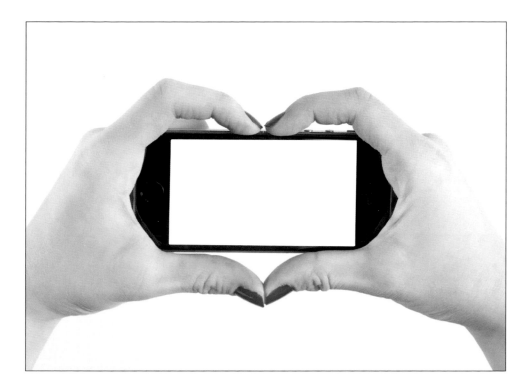

without your partner hearing (for what my bestie Katie Mack calls, "stealth-urbating"), pick a toy that is known for its quiet vibrations.

- **Consider a hands-free toy.** *WeVibe and OhMiBod both make Bluetooth-enabled toys that can be controlled via an app on your partner's phone or tablet.*

Hack: Share a Secret Pinterest Board

Great sex—or just getting some to begin with—is all about building anticipation. You could leave your partner a sexy note, or send a sexy snapshot, but here's a unique idea: set up a super-sexy Pinterest board and share it only with your lover. This could include sexy photos, quotes, sex tips, and positions you'd like to try. Then, throughout the day, the two of you can sneak a peek and pin photos and suggestions, all for your partner's viewing pleasure.

Hack: Download Some Steamy Apps

Is that something sexy in your pocket? Why yes, yes it is. By that we mean your smart phone. A little simple sexting can go a long way, but now you've got a whole arsenal of heat-inducing apps at your disposal too. There are apps for sending seductive photos, apps for making role-play suggestions, apps for acting out sex scenes, apps that dish out sex positions, apps that run sex games you can play with your partner, and much, much more. If you're like many people, you probably call on the powers of the Internet for just about everything. Why not use it to meet your NSFW needs too?

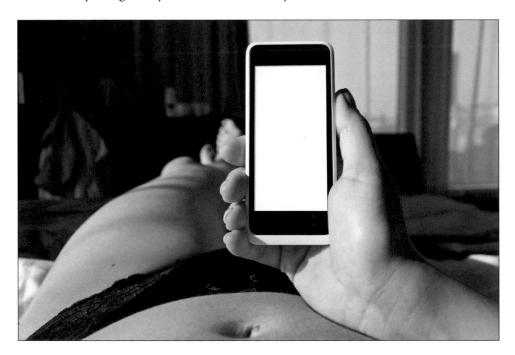

9. Sexual Self-Confidence Hacks

Believe it: There's something beautiful, stunning and commendable about everyone—even you. Easier said than done, right? If you're like most people, you're probably unhappy with your weight, or your shape or your nose or your feet. Although men suffer body image issues as well, the issue is rampant among women. In fact, when *Glamour* magazine surveyed more than 300 women of all shapes, sizes, and nationalities, only 3 percent admitted to loving their bodies. As for the remaining 97 percent, they admitted to having at least one "I hate my body" moment *every single day*. Similar surveys about men and body image are less available, but they do suggest that men are dissatisfied with their bodies as well.

Now, that's just plain sad. But beyond that, a lack of self-confidence also poses a danger to your health. Research from the University of British Columbia found that women who obsess over their bodies had elevated levels of stress hormones and were more likely to suffer from elevated blood pressure, lower bone density, higher levels of unhealthy belly fat, and even menstrual problems.

Now, just imagine what that emotional and physical fallout could do to your sex life! If you struggle to love your naked self, it will be much harder to truly share that body with your partner. Hey, it's really hard to orgasm when your brain's calculating how many calories you've eaten and whether you look fat against your new sheets. Low self-esteem can even dampen libido, which means you probably won't be having much sex at all.

So what can you do to learn to love yourself and the skin you're in, lumps, bumps, scars, and all? We've got a few handy hacks to help.

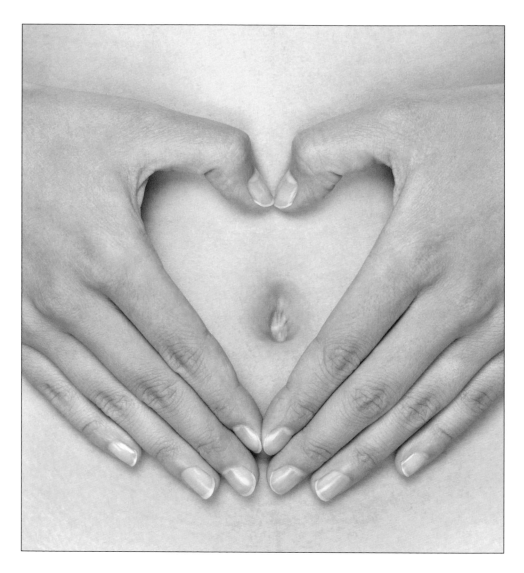

Hack: Send Yourself a Sweet Note

The first, best step to better sex is to love yourself, fully and completely. That's how you gain the confidence to ask for what you want—and to live in and enjoy the moment when your partner gets it just right. This sex hack comes from Jenne Davis, the head honcho over at clitical.com.

When it comes to the art of love, the one person women often forget about is themselves! One simple way to change this is by sending yourself a love letter once every couple of months.

Simply take a piece of paper and write down what you love about yourself! That's not your kids, not your house, but yourself. You might recognize that you are strong, or it might be a physical feature that you love about yourself, that you choose to write about. Don't worry about what you write, simply write. Now package it up in an envelope, add a stamp, and mail it to yourself. You can make the act of writing your own love letter as simple or as complex and fancy as you like.

I can pretty much guarantee that once you get that letter back, it will put a smile on your face when you open and read it. You can, of course, either tear up the letter or keep it at this point. I keep mine because they are a permanent reminder of how and what I loved about myself when I wrote the letter. They are fun to go back and read a year (or six) later!

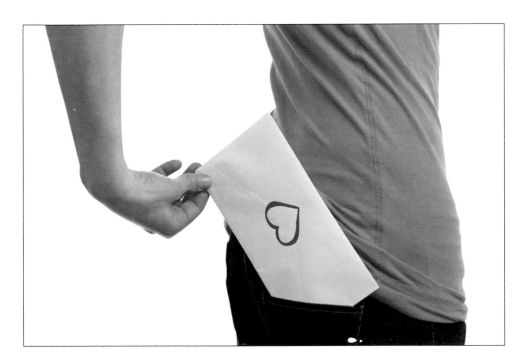

Hack: Make a Sex List to Get to Know What You'd Like in Bed

Think of the most confident person you know. Chances are, this person knows what they want in life—and isn't afraid to ask for it. The same goes for sex. Before you can be truly confident in your sexual self, you need to get to know your sexy side. This sex hack comes from Meg John Barker, author of *Rewriting the Rules*.

People often have a fixed idea about what sex is, and what they should be doing. Rather than doing what they might want to do, they often just do what they think is "proper sex." As a result, they don't get the chance to figure out what they actually really enjoy.

Spend at least ten minutes writing down all of the things that you could do, either by yourself or with another person, that you might find enjoyable sexually. Aim for at least twenty-five different things and make them quite specific. For example, instead of "oral sex," you might divide it into kissing, licking, sucking, etc., and be clear about which part of the body is receiving it. Try not to censor yourself at all, but just quickly scribble down everything you can think of without thinking too hard about it. Include everything, whether or not it's something you've done, or think you would enjoy. Allow yourself to think about all of the things that people commonly imagine when it comes to sex. Once you've done that, try to think of the less obvious kinds of things as well, like all the different ways you could touch or be touched, or non-touch-based things like sharing fantasies.

Once you've got a list of everything you can think of, you can go through it saying "yes," "no," or "maybe" about whether you'd like to do each of them. Some people give them a rating out of ten or add notes about how they'd like to do them or who with. This is something that you can keep for yourself or share with a partner, and invite them to do the same. Our lists change over time, so it's worth revisiting it every year or so. Also, saying "yes" on the list doesn't necessarily mean you'd want to do that every time, so it's still worth checking over with each other.

Hack: Set an Anti-Goal to Take the Pressure Off Something New

Sex can often become loaded with pressure because most of us are just so goal-oriented. We want to succeed at a new position, wow our partners on the first try, or just enjoy a great orgasm. The problem is, setting out with a goal in mind often backfires when it comes to enjoyment and pleasure. And isn't that the goal we should really have in mind? This hack suggests not just avoiding becoming fixated on a goal, but setting an anti-goal. It comes from gender-queer porn star Jiz Lee.

One of the biggest dilemmas in trying something sexual for the first time (especially if you're trying it with a partner) is the pressure to have it succeed. Sure, discussing what you want to do ahead of time is great, but if it leaves expectations . . . then that's just a recipe for disaster. There's a chance that in wanting so much for something to happen, you'll stop listening to the body's cues and sexual responses, making that very thing harder to accomplish.

The best rule when trying something new is to have an "anti-goal"—no, seriously. Go about trying something, but don't expect an outcome. Just try it for the sake of trying it. You'll have fun regardless. And who knows? You might surprise yourself in the process.

10. Sex Toy Hacks

Whether you play alone or with a partner, sex toys can totally change the game, often for the better. Now, we aren't going to come out and say that sex toys will save your sex life, but we also can't quite say they won't. After all, the health benefits of sex and masturbation are well documented, and sex toys are the perfect way to reconnect with a partner or yourself for some much-deserved pleasure and happiness. Plus, sex toys are all about fun (and they can be *a lot* of fun).

Want to bring playfulness and a sense of adventure to the bedroom? Bring some toys! Just be sure to share. These handy sex toy hacks are designed to help you wield your sex toys effectively, get off deliciously, and care for them properly so that you can do it all again tomorrow.

Hack: Be a Dildo Donna Reed

Maybe your house is a mess, but your sex toys probably aren't something you want to leave just lying around. You don't have to be a great housekeeper, but you can easily keep your sex toy collection as immaculate as the kitchens in those old movies, like actress Donna Reed did in *It's a Wonderful Life*. This sex hack from JoEllen Notte—aka The Redhead Bedhead (redheadbedhead. com)—will help you keep your play things in order and out of sight.

Love your sex toy collection but hate having to dig for your favorite when it's time for action? Simple household storage solutions will keep your stash organized and at the ready.

Hanging Shoe Organizer*: A standard over-the-door shoe rack has twenty-four pockets, each of which can easily accommodate a sex toy (more than* *one if necessary). This solution keeps your toys organized, relatively dust-free and, if you hang the organizer on the inside of your closet door, out of sight.*

Spice Rack: For a more visible solution, repurposed spice racks work beautifully. With so many design options, it is possible to find a rack for hanging flared-base dildos and butt plugs, or a rack that will support your fleet of vibrators as they stand like soldiers ready for action. There is even a rack that can hold dildos, vibrators, and plugs with their handles pointed out—ready for you to grab!

Tool Box: With their divided compartments and lift-out trays, tool boxes can be excellent sex toy storage solutions. They come in a wide array of sizes, from small enough to travel with to as large as a small bureau. What's more, many come with locks, so you don't have to worry about anyone getting into your stash.

Hack: Make Cleanup Easy by Putting Your Sex Toys in the Dishwasher

Believe it or not, you can wash silicone, glass, and metal sex toys in the dishwasher as long as they don't contain any mechanical parts (no vibrators!). Just place them in the top rack and run them on a gentle cycle, no soap. This is the simplest, easiest way to sterilize your sex toys and keep them squeaky clean. Whether you want to wash your dildos *with* your dishes is up to you.

Hack: Shake Things Up Inside with Ben Wa Balls

Ben Wa balls have a simple claim to fame: they made an appearance in a very famous and sexy scene involving a spanking in *Fifty Shades of Grey*. At their simplest, they are small, smooth, weighted balls that are inserted into the vagina, although more evolved versions include a string for removal. Because holding these puppies inside involves contracting the muscles inside the vagina, wearing them helps improve muscle tone. But they aren't

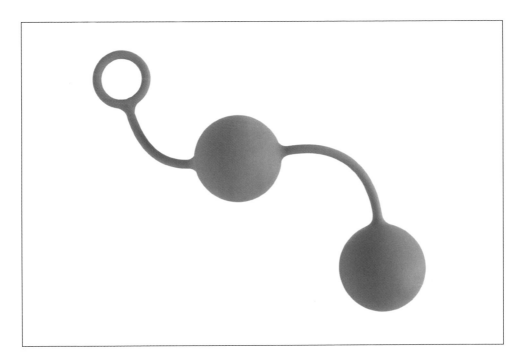

all work and no play; pairing them with a clitoral vibrator can produce a powerful orgasm. The external vibration causes the balls inside to vibrate, creating a whole new sensation.

Hack: Clean Up With Sex Toy Cleaning Spray

Keeping sex toys clean is important for your sexual health and the maintenance of your favorite bedtime play things. There are a lot of different methods and products out there for cleaning your toys, but a spray sex toy cleaner is a simple, easy method. This hack from Donna Turner, a writer for *LELO's Volonté* blog, adds a new twist.

Toy cleaning spray doesn't just keep your favorite pleasure products purring and pure. No, as well as helping to keep you safe and healthy, it can also be used to keep your windows, mirrors, and laptop screens gleaming. An alcohol-free

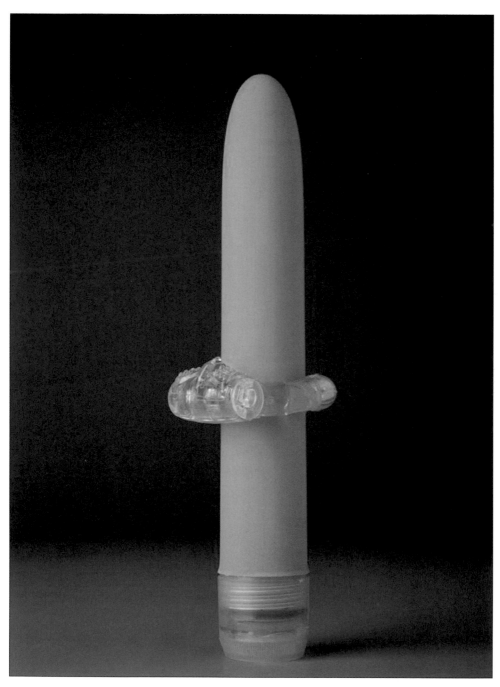

Source: Doc Johnson.

formula is (accidentally) great for cleaning any smooth surface, which is particularly useful if you enjoy using mirrors, or even webcams, as part of your play.

Hack: Create a "Recessionista Rabbit" Vibrator

There are soooo many sex toys out there, but which one to choose, especially when you have limited funds (and unlimited demands)? This fun, creative solution comes from Sunny Rodgers, the marketing director at Doc Johnson and radio co-host for "Ask the Doc" on Playboy Radio.

Everyone says we're coming out of our recession, but even if that is true, it won't stop us from loving coupons, sales, and especially hacks. Personally, sex toy hacks are my favorite. On top of saving my hard-earned money, I can justify buying more sex toys when I have multiple uses for them.

Best hack, hands down, is my Recessionista Rabbit. Rather than spending a hundred dollars or more on an actual Rabbit vibrator, I find a simple vibrator and a vibrating cock ring. Then I place the cock ring around the shaft of the vibe and use it as a clitoral stimulator. Clever! Plus, if you're like me, you'll appreciate the ability to slide the cock ring up and down so you can specifically target your hot spot in ways a regular Rabbit won't allow.

Hack: Enhance an Erection (and Orgasm!) With a Butt Plug

Butt plugs are a simple, less-intimidating intro to anal stimulation for both men and women, but they have an additional perk: because they put pressure on the male prostate, they can result in bigger, harder erections and a more intense orgasm. When using a butt plug, be sure to use lots of lube and insert slowly and carefully with gentle pressure.

Hack: Use a Wish List to Become a Smarter Sex Toy Shopper

Top quality sex toys are typically worth the extra cost, but that doesn't make them any easier to afford. Fortunately, this hack from sex positive blogger

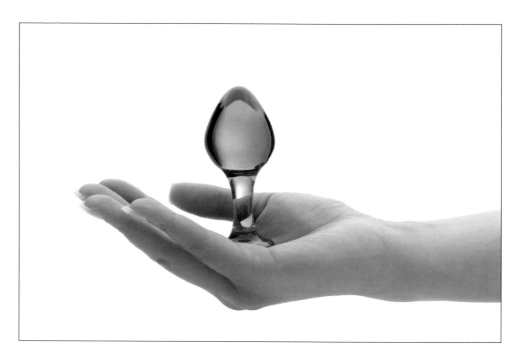

and sex toy reviewer Mandi at *EROcentric* (erocentric.wordpress.com) is here to help. Here's her advice on how to become a savvy sex toy shopper and score the goodies you want at a price that will leave you very satisfied indeed.

Sex toys can be a great way for individuals of any gender to learn about their bodies and explore pleasurable sensations. But high-quality sex toys can be expensive. When you consider that everyone's genital anatomy is unique and that toys are (almost always) non-returnable, deciding to purchase a sex toy can be rather scary. But there are ways to make your purchases less intimidating—and more affordable.

Much of my advice boils down to being a smart shopper. Don't buy toys on impulse. Do your research on the toy materials, the manufacturer's reputation, and the experience of sex toy reviewers online. Avoid companies that lie about their products and retail markets where sex toy counterfeits are rampant.

Create a wish list of the toys that seem like they'd be a good fit for you. Keep this list handy and be sure to check the clearance and sale sections of your favorite retailers often. In fact, you may even want to create a special bookmark folder in your Internet browser to speed up this process. Sign up for the electronic mailing lists of your favorite stores. This way you'll be notified of sales and you'll likely receive special coupon offers as well. If the items that you want still aren't being discounted, you can also try waiting for the major holiday sales (especially Valentine's Day, Black Friday/Cyber Monday, and Christmas).

Before you make your purchase, take an extra moment to look for additional purchasing incentives. Some companies may offer loyalty programs where you receive in-store credit for purchases you make or reviews that you write. You'll likely need to create an account, but this way your savings will stack up over time.

Oh, and the more you save, the more toys you can afford!

Hack: Judge a Dildo By Its Base

When you're picking out a dildo, chances are you're concentrating on the business end. You know, the one you'll actually be playing with. In fact, the base of a dildo is just as important, because it'll affect how you can use it. Want to use that dildo for anal play? Unless an embarrassing trip to the ER to retrieve said dildo is part of your fantasy, any dildos (or toys, for that matter) that you use for anal play must have a flared base. This ensures that the dildo won't, um, disappear. (As sex educators like to say, "without a base, without a trace.") The same goes for if you plan to use your dildo in a strap-on harness. Got it? Good. Now go forth and figure out what other features will turn you on.

Hack: Turn a Hair Tie Into a Cock Ring

Sex toys are great, but sometimes, when you're in a pinch, you need to improvise! There are all kinds of common items that can be perverted for your sexy pleasure. This handy hack comes from Lauren Palmer, the marketing manager for Revel Body vibrators. Just be sure that you never make any sort of cock ring too tight, and that you remove it as soon as the deed is done to avoid cutting off blood flow to the penis.

A thick hair tie can be used as a makeshift cock ring. Wrap it around the base of the shaft a couple times and it will slow the blood flow from the penis to help maintain an erection, just like a regular cock ring!

Hack: Want to Find Your G-Spot? Find the Right Toy First

The G-spot, or "Gräfenberg spot," is a bit of erectile tissue found between one and three inches inside the front wall of the vagina. Among scientists, there's been some debate about whether this fabled fun zone really exists, but for the women who've found theirs, there's no question: stimulation of the G-spot can produce deep, intense orgasms, perhaps even the best you've ever had. So how do you find this spot and connect with the pleasure it can produce? One of the best ways to start is to find a sex toy designed for G-spot stimulation. A vibrator or dildo designed for this purpose will have a pronounced or curved head, and will be firm rather than, um, *floppy*. You may also want to start with a simple clitoral vibrator to get warmed up. This helps send blood to the G-spot, which then engorges, swells, and becomes ready for more stimulation. Like all sexy fun, it'll probably take some experimenting to find out what floats your boat. Oh, and remember to relax and enjoy the ride. That'll help ensure a happy ending each and every time, whether it comes from your G-spot or not.

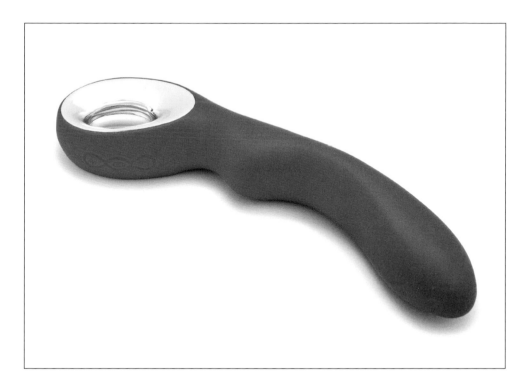

Hack: For a More Satisfying Vibrator, Look for Deep, Rumbly Vibration

If you're looking for a new vibrator, there are hundreds of options, but if it's pleasure you're after, it's best to pick a product that packs the right *kind* of punch. For most women, that means choosing a vibrator with deep, rumbly vibrations, instead of buzzy ones. What's the difference? Deep vibrations tend to come from higher-quality vibrators. They penetrate more deeply, stimulating the whole clitoris, which (did you know?!) is actually a vast structure of nerves that extend up into the pelvic region. Buzzy vibrations, on the other hand, are more likely to numb your nether regions, which kind of defeats the purpose. Read sex toy reviews to get a sense of which vibrators buzz just right, or try them out on your hand at your local sex toy retailer.

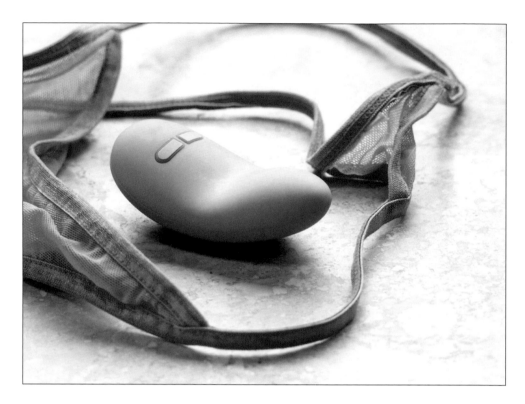

Hack: Use Salt to Quickly Clean Off Lube

The simplest tip out there for better sex is to use more lube. Slippery is fun. Period. Cleaning up said slippery? Well . . . maybe not. This simple clean-up hack comes from the *Crash Pad Series* porn star James Darling.

I once was told by a gay fisting enthusiast that you can easily remove water-based lube from your hands/arms/etc. by using salt! I would recommend not touching anyone's genitals immediately afterwards without washing your hands thoroughly but it's a neat trick to remove a lot of lube quickly! It's kind of like a naughtier version of a fancy exfoliating salt scrub.

Hack: Mix Silicone and Water-Based Lubes to Save a Silicone Sex Toy

Many of the latest, greatest sex toys are made of silicone, a soft, body-safe, and easy-to-sanitize material. The only catch? It breaks down if paired with silicone lubricant, which is often preferred for its long-lasting, ultra-smooth consistency. What to do? This sex hack comes from kink educator and pleasure artist Eve Minax.

Ever start playing around and realize you're using a silicone-based lube and now you want to use a silicone toy (they kill each other), doh! There's no time to run to the bathroom, wash everything off, etc., and besides, that would kill the mood. Assuming that you also have some water-based lube around, throw it in the mix! If you combine the two lubes at least 50/50, the solution should keep your toys safe and your play uninterrupted. This works both ways. So, if you want to add more viscosity, longevity, and safety to your play while using water-based lube, put in a bit of silicone, voila!

P.S.: Silicone lube can be hard to clean, so be sure to have some isopropyl alcohol around. It will make clean-up a snap!

Hack: Turn a Ping-Pong Paddle into a Custom Spanker

If a little pain is your pleasure of choice, you may want to bend over and give erotic spanking a try. A sexy spanking is a great way to inject some playful fun into an intimate experience and introduce an amazing array of new sensations. Not sure that spanking's for you? Professional sex, intimacy, and relationship coach Marla Renee Stewart (reneestewart.com) has a hack that'll help you enjoy a good spanking—without having to invest in a fancy sex toy.

Some of the best whips and paddles can be hundreds of dollars. If you don't have that kind of money, it's best to try to find some household products that

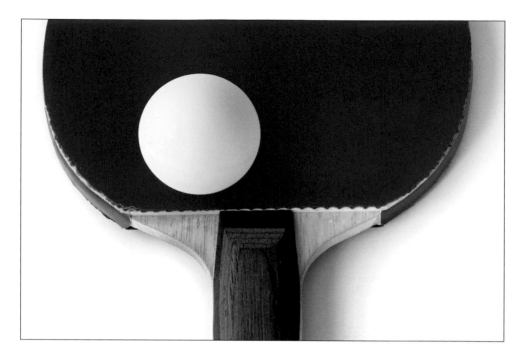

can strike your fancy (literally!). Most people use wooden spatulas or spoons, but if you want to take it a step further and you have an extra $10 in your pocket, you can purchase a basic ping-pong racket and make your own custom-signature spanking paddle!

Simply print out the mirror image of what you want your mark to look like, cut out the outline, trace it on your paddle, and then proceed to carve your design into the paddle with a box cutter or something similar. And then, voila! You have a brand new, customized paddle. Now all you need is a partner who's eager to bear your mark!

Hack: Shield a Sensitive Clitoris With a Towel or Washcloth

Genitalia are like snowflakes: each and every one is unique. That means that while some women need a jackhammer of a vibrator to get off, others cringe at too much stimulation. If your vibrator seems too intense, don't give up on it. Just put a towel or wash cloth between you and your toy. For many people this can mean the difference between cringing and coming.

Hack: Use Lube to Tame Flyaways

Once all is said and everyone is done, it might be time for a little freshening up. Lube to the rescue! This handy hack comes from Sunny Rodgers, the marketing director at Doc Johnson and radio co-host for "Ask the Doc" on Playboy Radio.

You've seen those expensive hair oils that banish flyaways—the ones with price tags that make you cringe. Now you'll be able to afford Starbucks and have ravishing hair! Silicone lubricant is perfect for keeping your hair soft, silky, and sleek. A dime-sized dab in the palm of your hand is all you need. Just rub through the ends of your hair for a polished look.

Hack: Use Flavored Lubricant to Create a Sensual Trail for Your Partner to Follow

Lubricant is often described in pretty clinical terms. It's marketed for "increasing comfort" and "reducing friction." It's great at both, but we think it can also be just for fun, especially when you're talking about flavored lubes. This sex hack comes from the president, CEO, and editor in chief of the sassy sex blog, *Slutty Girl Problems* (sluttygirlproblems.com).

Lubricant can of course make sex more comfortable, but it can also be used in much more interesting ways to heighten your sexual routine, especially when you bring flavors into the mix. It's a sexy, fun, and simple way to shake things up—and can easily be introduced to a new or old partner without the cost or possible intimidation of a whirring or buzzing toy. Don't let old misconceptions fool you—it's not just for oral sex! You can use flavored lube all over your body, in many ways, to add a little excitement to your romp.

Aside from flavoring your nether regions, you can trace a thin line of flavored lube across your intimate erogenous zones, like your nipples, collar bone, and inner thighs, and encourage your partner to lick or suck it off. Create a sensual trail to your hottest pleasure zones, or rub in the lube and ask your partner to simply follow the taste. If that's jumping the gun, try simply putting a little lube on your finger and having your partner suck it off, or vice versa! You'd be surprised how sensual this simple and seductive move is. Experiment with different flavors, and have your partner guess which flavor is in which place on your body. Don't worry, you're allowed to go back for seconds!

Hack: Use a Condom to Make Any Toy Waterproof

Bath time has never been more fun thanks to the increasing number of fully waterproof sex toys. But what if your very favorite vibe just isn't up to the task? Here's a hack from Sunny Rodgers, the marketing director at Doc Johnson and radio co-host for "Ask the Doc" on Playboy Radio.

How many times have you wished your toy was waterproof? Really waterproof? Not a good thing to ponder if it's a toy you really love and don't want to send to a watery grave. If you can relate, then I have a hack just for you! Place your vibrator inside a condom and tie a knot in the end. Now you can enjoy vibrations in the tub without worry.

Hack: Tease Your Partner With a Remote-Controlled Vibrator

Imagine if your partner could deliver orgasmic pleasure anytime, anywhere, at the press of a button. Actually . . . they can. Pretty sexy, right? There are a number of remote-controlled vibrators out there that allow one partner to cede control in exchange for pleasure. These vibes can be quite comfortable and discreet, so whether you play at home or in public, keeping your pleasure under wraps is half the fun.

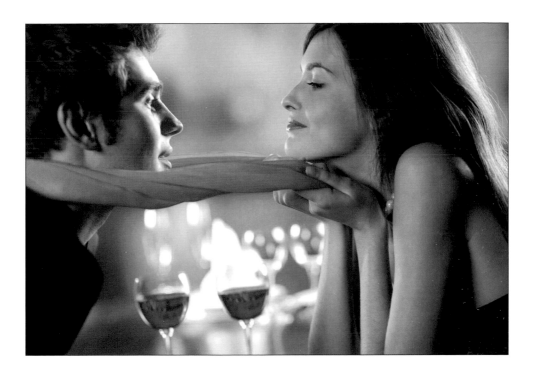

11. Kinky Sex Hacks

Think back to the days before you'd ever had sex. You were probably a little nervous about it. A little excited. A little afraid. And, if you were a normal teenager, you undoubtedly spent a whole lot of time wondering what it would be like. If you've never ventured beyond standard missionary position, or tied up a partner, or enjoyed a good spanking, trying something new—and a little kinky—is a little like being a virgin all over again. There's some apprehension—and a whole lot of excitement.

So what does kinky mean, anyway? In a general sense, kinky means engaging in activities that are a little taboo, or outside the boundaries of

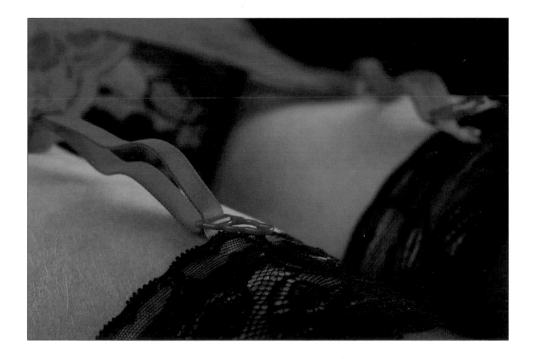

what some might consider socially acceptable. Sounds pretty fuzzy, right? The real answer is a lot more straightforward: you decide what kinky means for you. In other words, it's anything that pushes *your* limits. For some, that might mean a new sex position, or a pair of fuzzy handcuffs. For others, kinky might mean heavy bondage, multiple partners, or aggressive-looking sex toys. No matter what you choose, it's kinky because it excites you, pushes your boundaries, and turns you on.

Research shows that the more types of sexual activities a woman engages in, the more likely she is to orgasm. And, while there's no data to prove it, we can only imagine that guys like spicing things up too! Plus, discussing what sorts of things might turn you on can help intensify the connection between partners, while actually doing some of those things can really help boost a couple's sexual satisfaction.

Want to get your kink on but not sure where to start? Here are some hacks to help you take your sex life from nice to naughty.

Hack: Create a Kinky Sex List to Find Your Favorite Kinks

The key to great sex isn't in a certain position, or technique, or even in more foreplay. It's simpler that all of that. The key to sexual satisfaction is in learning how to communicate with your partner. Sounds kinda simple, right? Unfortunately, for many people, talking about sex is a lot like performing a complicated and difficult sex position: it's so overwhelming and intimidating and just, well, *hard,* that it's easy to skip right over it. The problem is, if your partner doesn't know what you want, you probably aren't going to get it. And that sucks.

One simple way to open the lines of sexual communication with a partner is to create a sex list. This is a big old list of lots of different sexual activities, with columns for "yes," "no," and "maybe" beside each one. You can find many versions of such a list online, or create your own. Print out copies for both you and your partner, so that you can each fill out the list on your own. Now comes the fun part: discussing and comparing your list with your partner. This will help you get to know your partner better—and give you both a wide variety of new and adventurous things to try out on each other. Plus, reading your lists makes for great foreplay.

Hack: Challenge Your Partner to a Sexual Wrestling Match

Like it rough? Jon Pressick, sex blogger, writer, and host of "Sex City" radio in Toronto, has a fun and creative hack for getting physical.

I grew up watching wrestling. I mean, what's not to like? Sweaty bodies pressed together in skimpy outfits . . . Oh, yeah.

Later in life, having acquired a definite interest in pain play and body thumping, I brought my early enjoyment of a little physical takedown into the bedroom, which led to a rather hot session of sexual wrestling.

For those who have explored BDSM, this is a new twist on many old favorites—with the addition of unpredictability. Before you start, everyone

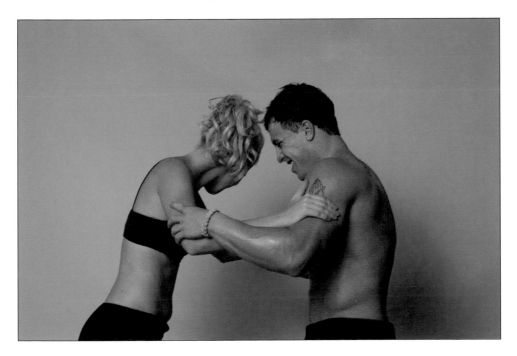

should be on board with boundaries and safety. Wrestling can be danger-
ous—even if you both try really hard to only hurt each other in the good way.
Establish a safe word so that your partner knows when to stop a hold or move
that goes beyond your comfort threshold.

Once "the rules" have been established, go at it!

Sexy wrestling can incorporate so many different sensual elements. There
can be slapping, spanking, tickling, or holding down. You can get more involved
and include humiliation and degradation. One person can take on a submis-
sive role while the other maintains dominance. Or it can be a free-for-all where
each of you is trying your damnedest to pin the other(s) down for a three count.
Blood will be pumping and skin will be teased. The tension of bodies in combat
is as challenging and exhilarating as it is sexy.

Hack: Play Pleasure Spoons

We often think about sex in terms of physical touch, but sensation play
involves arousing a partner via a variety of senses and creating different sensations. Temperature play is a great entry point to kinkier sensation play,
and often involves the use of hot or cold to awaken the skin's receptors. For
a simple take on sensation play, try placing a couple of spoons in the freezer,
and running a couple of others under hot water. Then alternate rubbing and
caressing your partner's body, allowing them to experience the chill, warmth,
and goose bumps that come from switching between the two. Electric!

Hack: Hire a "Cruise Director" to Coordinate Group Sex

Most people would consider group sex to be pretty kinky, but according
to research published by Bernice Kanner in 2004, 70 percent of people in
the United States have fantasized about it—and half of those have followed
through. As you might imagine, though, adding more people to the mix
can make things a little more complicated. This sex hack from dating coach
and sex educator Rebecca Hiles (friskyfairy.com) is designed to help ensure
everyone has a good time.

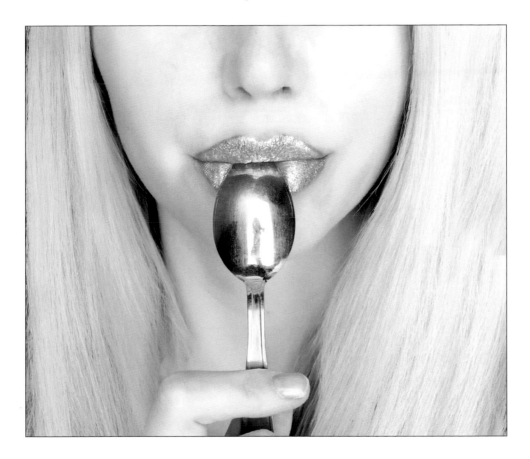

Group sex can be really awesome and also really scary, but there are three things that can absolutely help make the encounter run smoothly during the act. The first is to nominate a "cruise director." This person is your head coach, your stage manager, your master chef. This is the person who, if everyone else is feeling shy, is going to suggest positions, is going to move bodies, and will generally help coordinate a group of people who might otherwise feel incredibly awkward in a group sex situation. The second is to be prepared. Nothing is more of a pain than when you get to a group sex situation only to find that no one brought lube, condoms, toys, anything. It's better to be over prepared than under prepared. Finally, the best hack for a group sex situation is to

bring snacks! Bringing water to a group setting is excellent because people can really burn through bodily fluids during sex. It's important to stay hydrated! Also, having snacks around (my favorites are cupcakes and granola bars) means that anyone who needs a second to compose themselves, if they're feeling overwhelmed or anxious, can take a moment and have a snack without changing the dynamic but also still be a part of the energy during group play.

Hack: Practice Your Spanking on a Pillow

If a little pain is your pleasure of choice, you may want to bend over and give spanking a try—or deliver a swat or two to your partner. Because the buttocks are fleshy and fatty, it takes plenty of pressure to fire up this erogenous zone and bring on pleasurable sensations. That being said, not all spanking tips are created equal. A little experimentation will help you and your partner figure out what's best. The first step, however, is to test your aim. You want to aim your spanking at the fleshiest part of the buttocks; a whack around the tail bone or hip bones can be unpleasantly painful and even leave bruises. So, whether you're using your hand or some other implement of your choice, test out your aim and pressure on a pillow before delivering blows to your partner. Whether your partner is hankering for a little or a lot of pain, practice makes perfect!

Hack: Pervert Common, Inexpensive Household Items for Your Own Pleasure

Hankering to assemble a collection of kinky things, but can't afford all the leather and stainless steel your little heart desires? Fortunately, hardware, kitchen, and discount retail shops abound with bondage gear for the budget-conscious kinkster. This hack comes from professional Dominatrix and women's sexual wellness coach Mona Darling.

In the '90s when I started down the winding path that would lead me to a career as a successful professional Dominatrix, kinky toys were hard to find and expensive. I was a college student surviving on ramen, so I learned how to shop the hardware store, the kitchen section of Target, and the local thrift shop for what I needed. Now it's easy to find affordable toys, but there are still times when you either don't want to have obvious stuff lying around for parents or roommates to find, or a pile of kinky toys left for your heirs.

And sometimes it's just fun to shop Target and see what pervertables you can spot.

Some stuff is obvious. Wooden spoons make great paddles. A bar of soap is always good for a humiliation scene. Clips and clothespins can make great clamps (just be sure to test them for safety). Some other ideas:

- *Big, wide bag clips make awesome cock and ball restraints.*
- *A butter knife or fondue fork kept in the freezer is great for sensation play.*
- *And while you are in there, grab some ice cubes. They make great anal beads.*
- *Shoelaces have been spotted in more than one toy bag, and are the perfect length for cock-and-ball restraint. Add a second shoelace and you have a fashionable cock leash.*
- *Leather belts, scarves, and ties are great for restraints. Leather belts are also good for smacking unruly submissives. Consensually, of course!*
- *Fishing weights are great for ball stretching.*
- *Strips of gauze are great for making a quick, easy, and disposable hood.*
- *Resistance bands can make great cock-and-ball torture wraps.*
- *Plastic wrap—especially the stuff you get on a roller from the moving store—makes a pretty unbeatable mummification wrap.*
- *Paint stirrers make great paddles.*
- *Pretty much everything in the pink aisle at your local toy store is good for age play.*
- *Duct tape. What isn't it good for?*

This is just a quick list to start you looking for your own pervertables. Trust me, they are all around you waiting to be enjoyed with a snicker and a wink. No matter what you are playing with, always stick to your basic BDSM safety principles, and always discuss limits and get consent before you play. Oh, and never stick anything in the butt that doesn't have a flared base or something attached to it. Otherwise, you may be in for some very humiliating public medical play.

Hack: Make Your Own Harness Using a Pair of Underwear

Strap-on sex is gaining traction among people of all different genders and sexual orientations. But whether you're looking for girl-on-girl fun or bend-over-boyfriend action, you'll need a harness. There's a huge range of toys and products in this category, from rough-and-tumble leather harnesses to sweet and flirty silk briefs. But here's a little hack for those who want a little strap-on fun without having to make a big investment: make your own harness. Find a tight-fitting pair of underwear made of a sturdy fabric. Then, cut a hole in the front of your briefs where you'd like the dildo to sit. (Note that most people like to wear their dildos against the center of the pubic mound.) For best results, sew a rubber ring into the fabric to hold your dildo in place. Voila. You now have a cute, comfortable harness for a fraction of the cost!

Hack: Switch Things Up to Fortify a Flagging Erection

If all the ads for erectile dysfunction drugs are any indication, many men are very keen to keep their members at full mast. Unfortunately, drug-induced hard-ons aren't for everyone, and may even have serious side effects. This hack from sex writer, educator, and speaker Walker Thornton (walkerthornton.com) provides some tips on how to keep blood flowing in the right direction without having to resort to drugs.

Erectile difficulties occur more frequently as men age, but a weakened erection does not have to signal the end of sex. If he starts to lose his erection during sex,

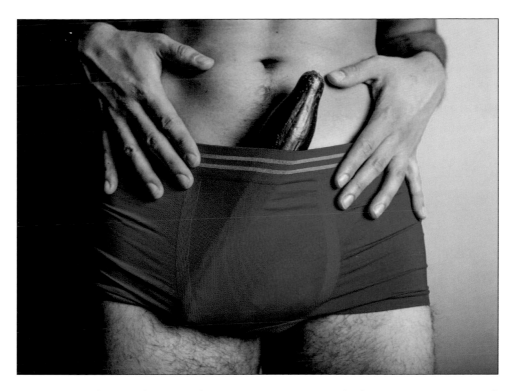

you can easily switch to another activity. For example, begin to caress or suck on his penis, or use your hands to see if you can increase his excitement and make his penis harder. If that doesn't work, stop focusing on his penis and move to other types of stimulation for a while—kissing or caressing.

Don't view his erectile issues as a failure, that's a mood killer. Instead, find other ways to pleasure each other. Give him a blowjob or use a vibrator on his penis or his testicles.

Just be sure to ask first and check to make sure the intensity is right. He might enjoy having you lube him up and straddle him, while giving him a hand job. Men are visual, so this position allows him to see and touch you while enjoying what you're doing.

There are several ways both of you can find sexual satisfaction—all fun and equally pleasurable—when erectile issues make vaginal penetration diffi-cult. It's as simple as redefining what sexual pleasure means to you.

Hack: Assemble an Aftercare Preparedness Kit

If you're into BDSM, you know it can be intense (in a good way!). And while many people like a good cuddle after sex, BDSM practitioners tend to take that concept a little further with what's called "aftercare," or taking care of a partner after playing out an exhilarating and exhausting scene. Aftercare can be performed in a lot of ways and depends on individual preferences, but this handy hack from Mandi, a sex-positive blogger and sex toy reviewer at *EROcentric* (erocentric.wordpress.com), encourages pre-pleasure preparedness.

Endorphins and arousal are a heady mixture, capable of creating very intense sexual experiences and even momentarily removing an individual from complete conscious awareness. Those in the BDSM community often cherish this powerful aspect of sexuality, but they also recognize that the ensuing comedown may cause physical, mental, and/or emotional exhaustion. Limits may have been pushed, role-played humiliation may require positive affirmations, and minor physical injuries may need to be attended to during what is called "aftercare."

Before starting a scene, it is important that you are prepared to provide proper aftercare when the need arises. To accomplish this, you should first talk to your partner about the concept of aftercare and discover what calms and relaxes them.

During this discussion, make sure that you consider a wide variety of options, targeting both physical and mental/emotional comfort.

Prepare a special "aftercare bag" for the unique needs of your partner. Include sensual relaxation materials such as candles/incense and a musical CD or playlist. Also consider any physical needs that your partner might have after a long, intense scene. Depending on the temperature of the play space, a small fan or a blanket may help to keep your partner comfortable. A beverage and snack may also be wonderfully refreshing.

Of course, an aftercare bag wouldn't be complete without a few medical supplies, just to be safe. You should always have a pair of safety scissors for quick and careful removal of any bonds. A basic first aid kit can also come in handy for minor abrasions.

Last, but certainly not least, be prepared to provide one-on-one emotional support for your partner, if that is something they desire. Cuddles and quiet, calming affirmations can play a very important role in the aftercare process.

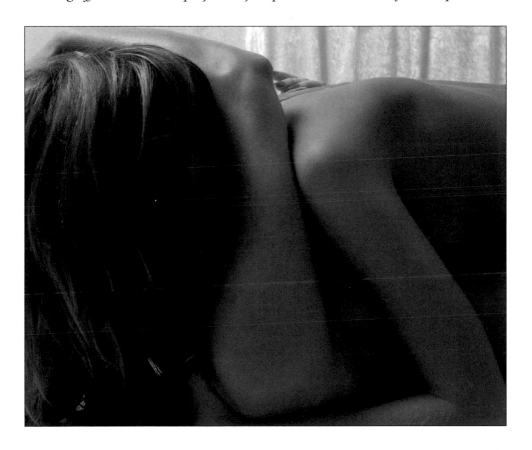

12. Climax Hacks

Type the word "orgasm" into any search engine and you'll get about seventy million results, most of which are articles on how to have more, bigger, better, longer, deeper, more explosive orgasms. Orgasm is seen as the coup d'état of sex, the apogee that concludes a successful sexual encounter. Now, we'd never knock a great orgasm, if you can get one, but for many people reaching the very best, most satisfying climax takes a lot more finesse than those brash, over-the-top magazine covers imply at the grocery store checkout line. In fact, the best lovers have a basic understanding of sexual anatomy, are in tune with their lovers' physical cues, and are eager to please.

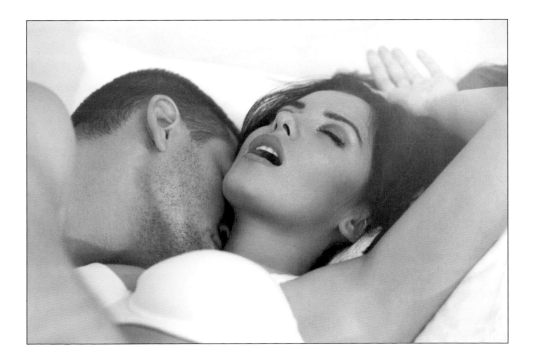

To have all of those skills, well, you've got to do some homework (it'll be fun though, promise!).

So why is that we're so obsessed with the Big O? Well, for a start, there's almost nothing like it, physiologically speaking. Orgasms are a full-body experience that include rhythmic muscle contractions, faster heart rate and breathing, raised blood pressure, and major activation of the brain's pleasure centers. In fact, an orgasm activates almost every part of the brain. Now that's some mind-blowing stuff. No matter what kind of sex you're having or who you're having it with, we're all seeking the same thing: satisfying sexual pleasure. Here are some hacks to help you get to the finish line.

Hack: Use a Rich Lube to Slow Down an Orgasm

A quickie can be a beautiful thing, but sometimes it pays to take your time and really savor a sexual experience. This sex hack from erotica author and sex blogger Kayla Lords (kaylalords.com) is all about slowing things down.

Any woman who masturbates often enough may eventually experience their own version of a quickie. You know what your body wants and needs, and it takes no time at all to get there. If you have a sensitive clit that allows quick orgasms (no really, they exist!), sex and masturbation can become a two-minute wham-bam-thank-you-for-nothing-ma'am.

Fortunately, there is a way to help desensitize your clit momentarily and slow down your orgasms so you can enjoy the build-up of tingles, pressure, and pleasure that comes from a slow-building, knock-your-socks-off orgasm: use a cream-based lubricant when you masturbate or during sexy playtime. These thicker lubes can act as a barrier between your body and the stimulation you're receiving, letting you enjoy your playtime a little bit longer.

For those that can and do have multiple orgasms from clitoral stimulation, the lube comes in handy when your clit is screaming no, but you aren't quite ready to be done yet. Plenty of people love watching multiple orgasms in action, but sometimes the body can't handle it. A good, thick lubricant helps. Bonus:

you'll stay nice and moist between orgasms, even if you need to take a break—or a nap—to recover.

Hack: Just Stop

Orgasm feels so good it's easy to race to the finish line. Try this instead: When you feel yourself reaching the brink, just stop. Take a few deep breaths, and take some time to kiss and pleasure your partner. Not only will this help you reconnect with your body, but you'll also extend your time together and increase your chances of having a bigger, better orgasm.

Hack: Engage Your Pelvic Floor Muscles to Increase the Chances of "Squirting"

A squirting orgasm is often considered a crowning sexual achievement for those who are playing with G-spot stimulation. Squirting, the expulsion of female ejaculatory fluid before or during orgasm, can be pleasurable, empowering, and visually impressive. And, while it isn't anatomically possible for everyone, many people hold it as a sexual goal. Hey, it's worth a try! Most people find that vigorous G-spot stimulation is what helps get them there, perhaps combined with clitoral stimulation. But here's one extra tip: As you approach orgasm, try bearing down on your pelvic floor muscles, producing a sensation of "pushing out" using the muscles around your vagina. This encourages fluid expulsion.

Hack: Hold Your Breath to Shut Out Annoying Distractions

Most men have a distinct sexual superpower: the ability to shut out the rest of the world when it's time for sex. Women? Not so much. Many report being distracted during sex. Needless to say, running through your to-do list while you're trying to get off doesn't enhance the experience. This sex hack from BDSM/sex educator and adult industry consultant Ken Melvoin-Berg can help a distracted partner get back to living in the moment.

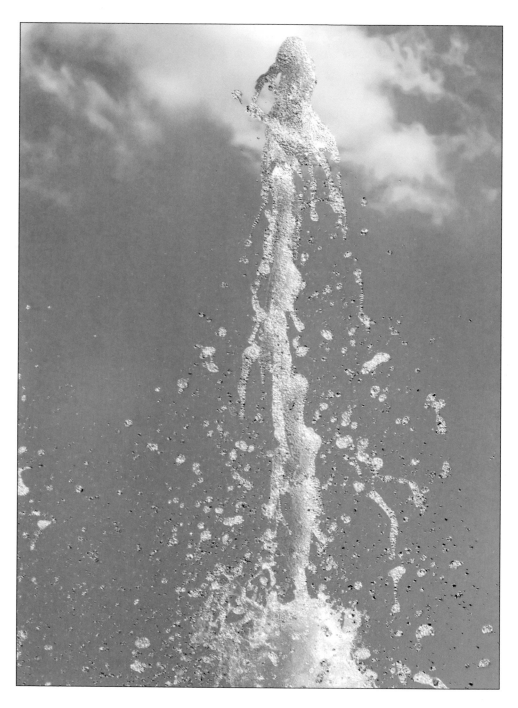

Occasionally a partner is distracted while having sex. Things like kids or dogs or even construction noise can be very distracting. One sex hack I use is breath control. When my partner is close to climax but seems distracted, I tell her to hold her breath. I count down from twenty to one and by the time one arrives, she is focusing on her breathing and not the distraction. Sploosh!

Hack: Squeeze Your Kegels for a Bigger, Better Climax

For anyone who lives or just dabbles in the BDSM word of power exchanges, kinky play, and Dominance and submission (D/s), at some point you may play with orgasm control. Controlled orgasms come in a few forms: forced orgasm, denied orgasm, and edging. This is a challenge because our bodies want to find their way to the pleasure zone as quickly as possible. This sex hack from sex blogger and erotica writer Kayla Lords (kaylalords.com) includes a simple trick for holding back a climax—for maximum impact.

Edging is the practice of being brought to the brink of a climax and then stopping the impending orgasm in its tracks, just before you go over the edge. I'm edged quite often in my relationship, and I've been told I must have such willpower and self-control. Not at all. I just figured out a trick that works!

If you need to stop your climax, squeeze your Kegel muscles. It sounds crazy, but squeezing the muscles that help you prevent urination can also help you prevent orgasm. You'll still feel the pleasure/torture of the continued stimulation making you desperate for an orgasm, but you should be able to hold it at bay.

As a woman, I can tell you it feels like my entire vagina opens and blossoms when I release the hold on those muscles and simply allow my body to do what it wants. Waiting also makes for a bigger, better orgasm.

Hack: Pulse Your Way to Pleasure

Orgasm involves a series of rhythmic contractions, or pulses. You can intensify this sensation for your partner by creating pulsations against various sweet spots as orgasm approaches. Place a finger or thumb over the clitoris and pulse gently. Press two fingers into the perineum (the area between the sex organs and the anus) and pulse firmly. Press a finger against the anal opening and pulse. Pinch a nipple and pulse. Press your palm into the vulva and pulse . . . you get the idea. Whichever area you choose, the brain and body will recall the pulsing spasms created by orgasm, thus bringing that orgasm nearer and making it into more of a full-body experience.

Hack: Use Rapid, Rhythmic Breaths to Increase Sexual Energy

In yoga it's called "breath of fire" and it can really heat things up in the bedroom and help you reach sexual nirvana. Here's how it works: As you approach orgasm, start making rapid, powerful exhalations through your nose, keeping your mouth closed. Keep your focus on the exhale and allow the inhalation to happen automatically. Keep your mouth closed. This shallow breathing heats

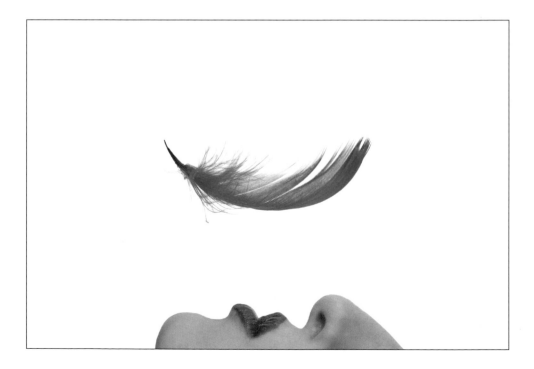

and oxygenates the body, a process that helps build sexual energy and elevate desire. It can also help keep you focused on what's happening in your body, allowing you to fully experience and enjoy the moment—and the big orgasm that this breathing technique can help produce.

Hack: Wear Socks for a Bigger, Better Orgasm (and Warmer Feet)

According to Planned Parenthood statistics, about 30 percent of women have trouble reaching orgasm when having sex; if we're talking vaginal intercourse, that number can be as high as 80 percent. There are so many tips out there about how to increase your odds, but here's the simplest one we've heard: wear socks. A study conducted at the University of Groningen in the Netherlands in 2005 found that 80 percent of women were able to achieve orgasm while wearing socks, while only 50 percent found their way to the Big O barefoot. According to the study's author, socks can help contribute

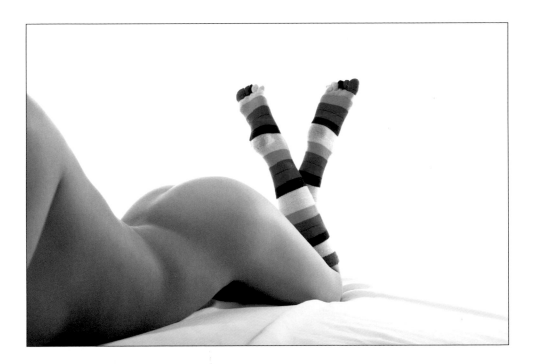

to a feeling of safety and comfort, thus deactivating the portions of the brain responsible for anxiety and fear. Forget lingerie—socks are the new sexy!

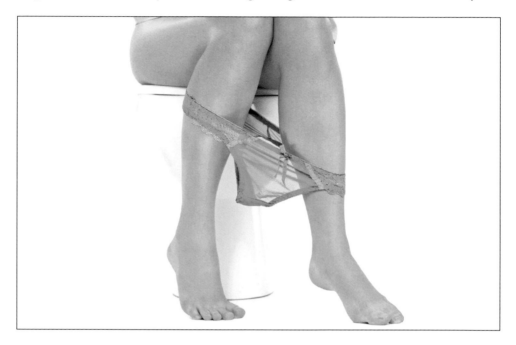

Hack: Hold It Until You're Done

There's nothing sexy about having to pee, but for many women a full bladder can trigger a more intense orgasm. This is because the fabled G-spot lies just behind the bladder, allowing a full bladder to add a little extra pressure. This hack is for ladies only though; for men, a full bladder can interfere with orgasm because releasing urine and ejaculation involve relaxation of the same sphincter.

Hack: Make Eye Contact to Improve the Odds of Simultaneous Orgasm

Coming together is a wonderful, albeit rare, kind of sexual crescendo. When it comes to heterosexual sex, men tend to become aroused and climax much more quickly than their female partners. But even in same-sex couples, individual differences in rates of arousal and ability to climax can make getting orgasmic response lined up very tricky. That said, when it does happen, it can be a beautiful thing. Along with slowing down, learning to control your sexual response and even having the faster partner masturbate before sex can help. You can also try making eye contact. This not only deepens your intimate connection with your partner, it's also a sexy form of communication that can help you gauge each other's pleasure.

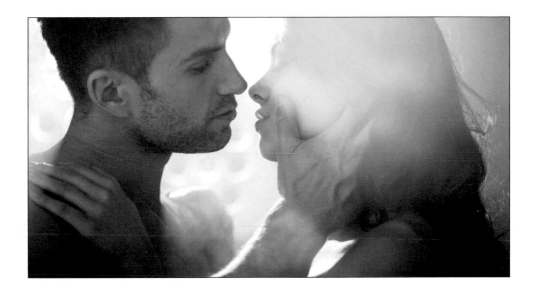